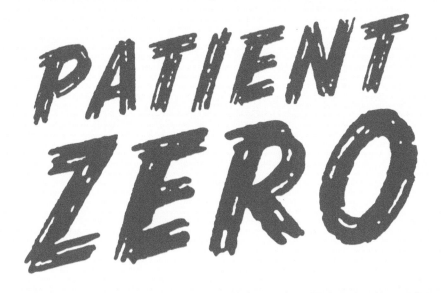

# PATIENT ZERO

---

## SOLVING THE MYSTERIES OF
## DEADLY EPIDEMICS

---

### MARILEE PETERS

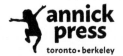

annick
press
toronto • berkeley

To Tom, Olivia, Jackson, and Frania—
a great bunch of people to spend a pandemic with.

Cover designed by Paul Covello
Designed by Elizabeth Whitehead
Edited by Catherine Marjoribanks
Proofread by Doeun Rivendell

The Publisher wishes to thank David Fisman, MD MPH FRCP(C), Professor, Dalla Lana School
of Public Health, University of Toronto for his expert review of the chapter on COVID-19.

Original edition by Marilee Peters published by Annick Press in 2014.

Annick Press Ltd.

We acknowledge the support of the Canada Council for the Arts and the Ontario Arts
Council, and the participation of the Government of Canada/la participation du
gouvernement du Canada for our publishing activities.

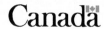 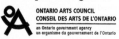

ONTARIO ARTS COUNCIL
CONSEIL DES ARTS DE L'ONTARIO
an Ontario government agency
un organisme du gouvernement de l'Ontario

**Library and Archives Canada Cataloguing in Publication**

Title: Patient zero : solving the mysteries of deadly epidemics / Marilee Peters.
Names: Peters, Marilee, 1968- author.
Description: Updated edition.
Identifiers: Canadiana (print) 20200327372 | Canadiana (ebook) 20200327380 | ISBN 9781773215167
(hardcover) | ISBN 9781773215150 (softcover) | ISBN 9781773215129 (HTML) | ISBN 9781773215136
(Kindle) | ISBN 9781773215266 (PDF)
Subjects: LCSH: Epidemics—History—Juvenile literature. | LCSH: Communicable diseases—History—
Juvenile literature.
Classification: LCC RA653.5.P48 2021 | DDC j614.4/9—dc23

Published in the U.S.A. by Annick Press (U.S.) Ltd.
Distributed in Canada by University of Toronto Press.
Distributed in the U.S.A. by Publishers Group West.

Printed in Canada

annickpress.com

Also available as an e-book. Please visit annickpress.com/ebooks for more details.

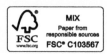

MIX
Paper from
responsible sources
FSC® C103567
www.fsc.org

# CONTENTS

# A NOTE ON THE SECOND EDITION

Thanks to Rick Wilks, Kaela Cadieux, and the team at Annick for making this update of *Patient Zero* possible, and in record time.

The updates to this book, including a brand-new chapter on the world's latest pandemic, were written in the spring of 2020 as the news media exploded daily with stories about the spread of COVID-19. While public health organizations, scientists, and government agencies around the world moved quickly to offer scientific information about this new virus and how to respond to it, it's also true that misinformation, myths, and plain old lies were spread as well, in both mainstream and social media.

Efforts to get reliable, helpful information to the public have been complicated by the fact that we are all still learning about COVID-19. As more information emerges, responsible scientists and public health officials have in some cases had to change their advice, and as a result some have been criticized for being "wrong." Like those scientists, I want to add a word of caution for readers: the information about COVID-19 that you will read in these pages is what was known by January 2021. In the months ahead, we will undoubtedly learn more, and some of what we think now about the virus may change. To some extent, that's true of all the diseases in this book—science never stands still, and there are always new discoveries to be made.

In some places, I have quoted directly from letters, reports, and journals of the people involved in treating or investigating the epidemics covered in this book. While their spelling has been modernized, their thoughts and ways of expressing them have not. In other cases, I have created dialogue to bring characters and stories to life, but always closely following the historical record.

# INTRODUCTION

# DISEASE DETECTIVES ON THE CASE

"So, tell me, where were you on the night of the murder?"

In movies or TV, when a detective asks this question, they narrow their eyes and lean in close to the suspect, to see how they'll respond. The audience pays attention too. We know that question is a sign that the detective is close to cracking the case.

Sure enough, the suspect starts squirming. Sweat breaks out on their forehead. Their eyes dart around in panic as they search their memory—or try to come up with a good excuse. Unless the suspect has an air-tight alibi, the detective announces, "Case closed!" A few scenes later, we watch as a cell door slams shut, putting the criminal behind bars. As the credits roll, the detective heads off into the night, to solve the next case and keep the public safe.

Now, take that detective out of their trench coat and fedora and put them in a lab coat. Instead of a gun, give them a microscope and a computer. This time, the assignment isn't to track down an escaped convict with a grudge, or a deranged psychopath masquerading as a friendly neighbor, or any of the usual suspects. The murderer they're trying to identify is—a microbe.

This is a disease detective. Otherwise known as epidemiologists, these scientists are trained to solve medical mysteries and find the evidence needed to prevent the spread of disease and improve the public's health. Like police detectives, epidemiologists make a beeline for the "scene of the crime" when a disease first strikes, to search for clues that reveal how the outbreak started, how it is transmitted, what puts people at risk of getting sick, and how to stop or slow its spread.

Just like the hardboiled detectives in old movies, they talk to the victims, track down witnesses, ask lots of questions, sniff out facts that may have been overlooked, and then assemble their case. In addition to these tried-and-true detective techniques, they also take advantage of the latest technologies and use their scientific skills and know-how to understand how diseases spread and to protect our health.

The investigation into an outbreak starts with the first patient who shows up at their doctor's office or local hospital with an illness. While epidemiologists call this first patient the "index case," in the media and popular culture this person is often referred to as "patient zero." (Spoiler alert: to find out how "patient zero" became a popular term for the first known case in an outbreak, flip to chapter 7.) Starting from this first case, epidemiologists trace the infection's spread. They look for clues that help them understand the factors that contribute to the transmission of the disease.

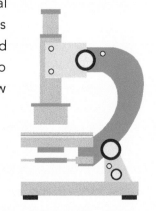

# TOOLS OF THE TRADE:
# THINK LIKE A MICROBE

Epidemiologists are up against tiny but powerful enemies: the microbes that make us sick. Although they are microscopic, they vastly outnumber us (there are as many *species* of microbes as there are stars in the galaxy!). Fighting this invisible army depends on understanding it.

To start with, not all microbes are bad guys. Microbes live all around us, and in us. Some make us sick, but many others—like the ones that live in our guts and help us digest our food—are important for our health.

Viruses are incredibly tiny microbes that can only survive inside the cells of other living things. A virus invades a host cell and takes it over, using the cell's energy to multiply itself and then releasing new viral particles that go on to infect more cells. Most viruses cause diseases in the host organism and have evolved ways of spreading to new hosts through the disease.

For example, influenza viruses make us cough and sneeze. Each time we do, we spread viruses in clouds of droplets, giving them a chance to find new homes in other humans. The cholera virus gives its unlucky hosts diarrhea, and the virus spreads to others when their waste finds its way into drinking water supplies. Sometimes—as with malaria and yellow fever—a virus will be in the host's bloodstream, and when a mosquito takes a bite of blood from one host and then bites another, the virus comes along for the ride, and now two people are infected. For an epidemiologist, knowing how a microbe spreads is key to understanding and stopping an outbreak of disease.

This means tracking down, one by one, everyone the infected person came into contact with. It takes patience and determination—and it also doesn't hurt to have charm and a sense of humor when you're asking people to try to remember everyone they might have coughed on recently!

Lots of the detective work of epidemiology happens at a local level, by knocking on doors and talking to people who may have been exposed to the disease. But epidemiologists also need to coordinate their disease-fighting efforts with other scientists, and with governments and public health agencies nationally and internationally. Today, a disease outbreak can spread around the world in just days, or even hours. To be prepared for that kind of global threat, modern epidemiology requires teamwork, cooperation, and endless tracking of information about health concerns from all nations. At public health agencies like the World Health Organization (WHO), the Centers for Disease Control and Prevention (CDC) in the United States, and the Public Health Agency of Canada (PHAC), epidemiologists are constantly scanning new reports from all around the world of unusual diseases, or new outbreaks of known diseases. They know that any one of them could be the next "Big One."

In December 2019, doctors in Wuhan, China, started seeing an increase in the numbers of patients with pneumonia. When they realized they might have an outbreak of a new disease on their hands, they notified the WHO, an agency of the United Nations that looks after international public health. Those pneumonia patients were the earliest victims of a virus that had jumped from an animal host to humans, triggering an epidemic that led to a global pandemic: COVID-19. "The Big One" had arrived.

COVID-19 turned 2020 into the year of the epidemiologist. Epidemiologists held news conferences, gave interviews, recorded podcasts, appeared in YouTube videos, and made animated visuals mapping the spread of the infection.

But epidemiology isn't all bright lights and glamour. The scientists who unraveled the medical mysteries behind the diseases covered in this book faced a terrifying prospect: they were tracking down infected patients, working in communities where disease was rampant and deadly, and risking their lives. They needed to be courageous and very determined—all too often, no one believed their crazy theories. They were ignored, laughed at, sometimes even fired from their jobs. But they kept searching for answers, putting together the puzzle pieces of these epidemics. Millions of people owe their lives to the work of these early epidemiologists. Thanks to their willingness to do the dangerous work of tracking diseases to their source, we now know how to prevent or cure some of history's most deadly diseases.

# A CORONAVIRUS CHEAT SHEET

Beginning early in 2020, we started hearing the messages on TV, on social media, and in our schools and our communities: "Save lives, #flattenthecurve," "We'll get through this together by staying apart," "#socialdistancing." The messages and hashtags are all public health advice drawn from epidemiological science. Here's a primer on some of the most-used terms.

**Contact tracing:** Methods that public health officials use to track the spread of the virus. Infected people are asked about their recent activities and to list others they have interacted with. Those people are contacted and told to stay home and to get care if they develop symptoms.

**Flattening the curve:** Slowing the spread of the virus so that fewer people need to seek treatment at the same time, by following practices such as social distancing, self-quarantine, hand-washing, etc.

**PPE:** Personal protective equipment such as gloves and masks, along with more specialized gear worn by health care workers, such as face shields, gowns, and foot covers.

**Self-isolation:** People who are infected with COVID-19 are required to stay at home and away from those who are not sick while they have active symptoms of the disease.

**Self-quarantine:** Staying at home, apart from others, for a period of time (usually 14 days) to see if illness develops. In some places, people are required to self-quarantine if they have been exposed to the coronavirus or if they have returned from an area with widespread transmission of the disease.

**Shelter-in-place:** Not quite as strict as a self-quarantine, this means to stay home, only leaving for essential reasons or to exercise.

**Social distancing:** Maintaining a physical distance from others that is greater than usual, and avoiding busy public places. Also sometimes called physical distancing, this reduces the chance of becoming infected.

# GET OUT YOUR EPI-DICTIONARY

Listening to the news about COVID-19 or any other emerging disease, you might start to wonder if epidemiologists have their own language. For instance, what's the difference between an "endemic disease" and an "epidemic"? What's worse, an "outbreak" or an "epidemic"? When does an "epidemic" become a "pandemic"?

**Endemic disease:** These are the diseases that are always around, the ones doctors expect to see year after year in particular areas of the world. Malaria is rarely seen in North America, but it is endemic to certain parts of Africa, where it occurs regularly.

**Outbreak:** When a relatively small number of people get sick with the same disease at around the same time, it's called an outbreak. An outbreak of disease could be triggered by a single event, like some undercooked hamburgers that send everyone at a family reunion to the hospital. Or an outbreak can happen when an endemic disease from one place turns up unexpectedly somewhere else. For instance, in 2019 someone with dengue fever visited Hawaii and was bitten by mosquitoes. Those mosquitoes transmitted the disease to other people in Hawaii, causing an outbreak.

**Epidemic:** An epidemic is an outbreak, multiplied. New cases are actively spreading, and the numbers of cases are higher than what is normally expected. When doctors start reporting an unusual number of patients with the same symptoms, public health authorities may declare that there is an epidemic underway. They'll alert the media so that people can take precautions against the disease.

**Pandemic:** If the epidemic can't be contained, it may become a pandemic—a global epidemic that infects a large number of people over a very wide area, in different countries and regions of the globe. The World Health Organization considers that w hen an epidemic is reported in three or more countries, it's officially a pandemic. One way to remember the difference between an epidemic and a pandemic is the *p*—a pandemic is an epidemic with a passport.

# CHAPTER 1

# A DEADLY YEAR

## THE GREAT PLAGUE OF LONDON, 1665

The rat looked dead. Goodwoman Phillips nudged it with her toe to be sure. It didn't move.

She bent down, pinched its tail between her thumb and forefinger, and lifted the rat up so it dangled limply before her face. "Come into my kitchen and die on my clean floor, will you?" she said menacingly to the little corpse. "We'll see about that, you dirty beast." Goodwoman noticed with disgust that fleas were still jumping in the rat's coarse black fur—it hadn't been dead for long. Probably frozen to death: the winter of 1665 was the coldest she could remember.

She opened the door and swung the rat by its tail, flinging it as far from the house as she could. It landed with a thud in the gutter. "Good riddance," thought Goodwoman Phillips. She wiped her hands on her skirt before heading inside to make breakfast.

She thought no more about the rat that day. She was a busy woman, with a husband and sons to feed. For a poor family like hers, living outside the walls of London in the rough-and-tumble parish of St. Giles in the Fields, food was often hard to come by. Worse, with this winter's dreadful cold, they needed more fuel than usual for the fire. Goodwoman feared that the extra expense would mean Christmas, not even a week away, would be a lean and dismal holiday this year.

Goodwoman Phillips was right to worry about Christmas. There would be no celebrating in her home. As that dark December day wore on, her head began aching, and pain grew in her back, arms, and legs until she could hardly stand. Then fever and chills set in. By evening she was forced to take to her bed. She lay in a daze, trying not to moan.

## SIGNS IN THE SKY

Day by day, Goodwoman Phillips got sicker. Her sons sat by her bedside in the evening, trying to distract her with the latest news from London. The whole city was buzzing with rumors about the comet that had been seen flaring across the heavens every clear night since November.

Many believed that the comet was a sign from God to England's king, Charles II, who had been on the throne for just four years. People remembered an old superstition that the crowning of a new king would be followed by plague. "These Blazing Stars Threaten the World with Famine, Plague, & Wars. To Princes, Death; to Kingdoms, many Crises; to all Estates, inevitable Losses!" was the dismal forecast of one popular astrologer.

As a fresh wave of fever shook Goodwoman Phillips, her sons crept away, leaving her to rest. Soon she was tossing in a restless, feverish sleep.

# HOUSE CALL

When Goodwoman Phillips opened her eyes next, it was light in the room. A tall man in a long coat was unpacking a leather satchel and laying out items along the wooden bench under the window. A cup, a cloth, a knife. Goodwoman realized at once who this man was and why he was there. A doctor!

"I'll not be bled." She tried for a firm, clear tone, but even to her own ears her voice was low and faltering. The doctor turned and looked at her calmly.

"Goody Phillips, your husband and sons have consulted me about your case. Bleeding will balance the humors within your body. It is for the best."

The doctor came closer. She could see the knife glinting in his hand. Then it was done, a smooth, quick cut on her arm. Blood dripped into the cup he held up. Her head thudded and the room seemed to lift and tilt, then spin.

"Fainted," said the doctor. "Not uncommon for one so far gone with fever. Let's hope this bloodletting was done in time."

Goodwoman Phillips didn't wake again. On Christmas Eve of 1664, she died, the first victim in an epidemic of plague that was to kill nearly one in five Londoners over the coming year.

## IT'S NOT FUNNY, IT'S HUMORAL

From ancient times until the 19th century, when a doctor told you your humors were out of balance, he didn't mean that there was something wrong with your funny bone. Humoral theory was one of the key principles in Western medicine.

According to this theory, first proposed by the doctors of ancient Greece, the human body contained four humors, or fluids: black bile (also known as melancholy), yellow or red bile, blood, and phlegm. Your health depended on maintaining the right humoral balance, or mix of fluids, inside your body. Curing disease was a matter of putting the humors back in balance. This is where the idea of bleeding patients came from.

## "GOD HAVE MERCY UPON US!"

A neighbor woman came that afternoon to wash the body and prepare it for burial. When the neighbor removed Goodwoman Phillips's nightdress, she gasped: large red rings had appeared on the dead woman's chest and back. Under her right arm was an ominous purple swelling.

"A buboe! Plague tokens!" whimpered the shaken woman. "Plain as my hand, these are the signs. This is a plague house. Oh, God have mercy on us!" She turned and fled down the stairs and out of the house.

Before long, there was a knocking at the door of the Phillipses' tiny house. The searcher had arrived. It was the searcher's duty to visit every house where a death occurred in St. Giles in the Fields, to examine the deceased and to report back to the parish clerk, who recorded the cause of death in the parish register.

All 119 London parishes kept registers of births and deaths, bulky volumes filled with line after line describing deaths from old age, accidents, and illnesses of every kind. Yet of all the ways to die in 1664, none was more feared than plague, for plague could spread through a neighborhood like fire. In a matter of weeks, plague could engulf a whole city, even a whole country.

The searcher for St. Giles in the Field was a shrunken, wrinkled old woman. She was desperately poor and spent every cent she had on ale at the inn. It was well known that she'd gladly take a coin or two should a family wish to have the cause of death changed in the report she delivered to the parish clerk. For a small tip, a suicide could become an "accident." Even plague could be registered as a simple fever. But the Phillips family had no money to offer her. Her sons had spent everything they had to bring the doctor in to bleed their mother.

The searcher peered down drunkenly at the body, then reeled away in alarm at the sight of the swollen lumps called buboes, proof that Goodwoman Phillips had died of the disease we now know as bubonic plague. She staggered off, returning later with men from the parish office, who began boarding up the doors and windows. The dead woman's family would not be allowed to leave their house for weeks, in case they spread plague to others.

Inside the darkened house, Goodman Phillips and his sons listened as nail after nail was pounded into the boards blocking their windows. Finally, the pounding was replaced by the softer sound of brushes. A huge red cross was painted on their door, and the words "God Have Mercy

Upon Us." Those signs let everyone in the neighborhood know that this house was cursed with the plague.

That Christmas Eve, all was silent in the Phillips house. Goodwoman's husband and sons could only wait and wonder: Which of them would be next?

Outside, their neighbors crossed the street to avoid walking past the boarded-up house, fearing that if they came too close, they would be contaminated with "plague seeds."

# THE FEAR BUILDS

A little more than a week after the death of Goodwoman Phillips, soon after New Year's, John Graunt stepped to the door of his London shop and tossed a coin to one of the ragged boys shivering in the frosty January air outside.

"Run and fetch me a copy of the Bills of Mortality. The first bill of the year was printed this morning, and I'm anxious to see it. You may find me in a generous mood to repay you for your speed." As he watched the boy disappear up the cobbled road, John considered how surprising it was that the Bills of Mortality, a page of statistics listing the week's births and deaths in each London parish, should have become so popular with readers. Each week in the coffeehouses and the taverns, conversation was sure to turn to the latest news in the bills—especially if there were any unusual deaths.

John Graunt always found the Bills of Mortality fascinating, but he'd heard that there was something he would find particularly interesting in this week's edition. And when the errand boy ran back with the page fluttering in his hands, it didn't take long for John to spot it: "Death by Plague—1."

London hadn't had an epidemic of plague for nearly 20 years. And plague usually struck in the hot months of summer, not in the midst of the coldest winter that anyone could remember. But all the same, John decided to keep a close eye on the bills over the next few months.

For the rest of that cold, dark winter, while all of London was watching the sky, John was scanning the lists of deaths, reading the signs there that told him an epidemic of plague was coming again.

# LOOKING FOR ANSWERS

As the owner of a popular haberdashery (a store selling cloth), John Graunt was an expert on everything from the coarsest cottons to the finest silks and velvets, along with buttons, thread, and ribbons in every color of the rainbow. But running a successful business wasn't enough to keep John's active mind occupied. He really wanted to make a name for himself as a scientist or a scholar. He'd always been fascinated with the weekly Bills of Mortality, and by the late 1650s he had saved several years' worth of the weekly statistics. John realized that those dusty stacks held a treasure trove of information.

As a businessman, he knew the value of having information about his customers. He needed to know approximately how many births to expect each year so that he could stock the right amount of delicate linen for christening robes. And by knowing how many deaths there might be in a year, he could have enough cloth for mourning clothes on hand. At the time, there was no source for this kind of data. John, like other shopkeepers, was forced to depend on his intuition and experience when ordering his stock. Yet since 1592, the weekly Bills of Mortality had been tracking these numbers, and more. By reading through all the bills and adding up the deaths and the births, John realized he would be able to work out annual averages, and perhaps find useful patterns.

He began to wonder what other uses there might be for information about birth and death rates in his city. Comparing the numbers of deaths and their causes from one year to another might reveal patterns not only in how many people were dying, but also why.

John Graunt decided that he had found the perfect subject for a scientific study.

## WHAT ABOUT DYING OF CURIOSITY?

Plague wasn't the only thing killing Londoners during the 17th century. The Bills of Mortality were full of unusual ways to die. Some that you are not likely to see in an obituary today include: "Stoppage in the Stomach," "Twisting of the Guts," "Eaten by Lice," and the mysterious "Horseshoe head."

## SUCCESS AT LAST

John Graunt collected all the Bills of Mortality from the past 60 years and studied them, looking for the secrets that they held about London life. In 1662, he published his findings in a short book with a long title: *Natural and political observations, mentioned in a following Index, and made upon the Bills of Mortality: With reference to the Government, Religion, Trade, Growth, Air, Diseases and the several changes of the said City.*

# BLAST FROM THE PAST

Many people have heard of the Black Death—the pandemic of plague in the Middle Ages that killed almost a third of the people in Europe. But the world has suffered through not just one but three plague pandemics.

The first is known as the Plague of Justinian. Named after the Roman emperor Justinian I, the disease first broke out in Constantinople (modern-day Istanbul, Turkey) in 541 CE. It swept through the city, killing up to 5,000 people a day, before going on to spread across Spain, Italy, Africa, and the Middle East. Over the next three years, it killed as many as 50 million people.

Afterward, plague outbreaks continued but didn't reach pandemic levels again until 1347, when traders and invading armies carried the disease into Europe. Whole villages were wiped out by the Black Death, crops went unharvested, and trade stopped. Some historians think one third of the population died in the pandemic. It took 200 years for the population to recover.

The next great pandemic of plague started in 1855 and lasted 100 years. Rats hiding in steamships carried the disease across the world, causing outbreaks in port cities on every continent. Over 15 million people died.

Will there be a fourth pandemic of plague? Its possible but unlikely. Plague can now be treated with antibiotics, and thanks to modern hygiene many cities are cleaner, with fewer rats.

His book was an instant hit, and in 1663 John was admitted to a very exclusive club of scientists: the Royal Society of London for Improving Natural Knowledge. Although John modestly described his accomplishment as just "shopkeeper's mathematics," he'd developed a method for predicting the arrival of a plague year. This was a tremendous scientific advance. For more than a century, the people of London had suffered regular epidemics of plague—one almost every 20 years. Tens of thousands had died, and the city's inhabitants lived in fear of the next outbreak.

By studying the Bills of Mortality, John realized that in the months leading up to an outbreak of plague, deaths from all causes were higher than usual. "Sickly years," he called them. The winter of 1664 was the start of a very sickly year in London. Goodwoman Phillips's death was the first one to be recorded as plague, but he was sure it wouldn't be the last.

## THE SICKLY YEAR THEORY

By watching the number of deaths closely and seeing as they began to rise each week, John Graunt was able to predict a plague epidemic. He looked at all deaths, not just from plague, because he knew the system for recording deaths in London wasn't very accurate.

Years before, King James I had ordered each London parish (the district surrounding a church) to begin keeping track of all the local births and deaths. Officials called parish clerks were in charge of the records. Since there weren't enough clerks to track down all the births and deaths in the crowded city, they depended on "searchers," like the one who visited Goodwoman Phillips's home, to collect the information they needed.

This system had a few problems. For one thing, the searchers had no medical background. When it wasn't clear what someone had died

# TOOL OF THE TRADE:
# DESCRIPTIVE EPIDEMIOLOGY

Epidemiology (pronounced epeh-dee-mee-ol-o-gy) is all about looking at the "big picture" of a disease outbreak. While physicians try to help individual patients get well, epidemiologists help to keep us from getting sick in the first place. To do this, they need to understand who is getting sick, what's causing the disease, and how it is spreading. Once they have that information, they can try to figure out how to stop the outbreak.

Most countries today keep track of deaths and any unusual cases of infectious diseases. In 1665, there was very little of this kind of information. John Graunt was the first person in England to realize that keeping accurate records of the number of people who died each year could help fight disease. His analysis of the Bills of Mortality for 1664 and 1665 is one of the earliest examples of what we now call "descriptive epidemiology." It is the first step in putting together the big picture of a disease outbreak.

For an epidemiologist, putting together that big picture means using data—lots of it—to describe the who, what, when, and where of the outbreak. The answers to these questions are clues to how and why the epidemic is spreading: information that they can use to fight the disease.

from, they had to guess. This led to some unusual entries in the Bills of Mortality, like "teeth," "pining," "evil," "fools etc.," and "found dead."

In addition, the searchers weren't paid much, so for the price of a drink and a few extra pennies, many searchers would agree to write down anything they were told. When someone had died of plague, their family would be eager to bribe the searcher to cover it up. Otherwise, the whole family would be shut up in the house, to prevent them from spreading "plague seeds." John Graunt estimated that up to 20 percent of plague deaths were recorded as something else in the Bills of Mortality.

The third problem was that the parish clerks only recorded the births and deaths of citizens who belonged to the official religion, the Church of England. This created big gaps in the official statistics because it left out other religious groups: Jews, Catholics, Quakers, and Non-Conformists.

There were a few more plague deaths in London through the rest of that cold winter, and as the weather warmed up, the numbers began to increase. In the first week of June, 43 deaths from plague were recorded—as many as there had been for the whole year up till then. The next week, there were 112. By fall that year, 7,000 people were dying each week. Plague had returned to London, with a vengeance.

Soon, anyone who could afford to leave the city began packing their bags.

John Graunt stayed where he was. He had his shop to look after, but more importantly he wanted to keep an eye on the information coming from the parishes each week. His theory about sickly years leading to plague years was being proven before his very eyes.

# THE STREETS ARE EMPTY

By mid-July, there were 1000 people dying in London each week. By September, it was up to 1000 a day. A Londoner named Samuel Pepys wrote in his diary, "But now, how few people I see, and those walking like people that have taken leave of the world."

Samuel was a successful businessman. But unlike most wealthy people, he didn't leave London during the plague. Instead, he stayed and recorded his impressions in his diary, which was published almost two centuries later. It is one of the most revealing records of what life was like for people in London during that terrible year.

In the fall, with plague raging across the city, Samuel wrote, "Lord, how empty the streets are, and melancholy, so many poor sick people in the streets, full of sores, and so many sad stories overheard as I walk, everybody talking of this dead, and that man sick, and so many in this place, and so many in that. And they tell me that in Westminster there is never a physician, and but one apothecary left, all being dead—but that there are great hopes of a great decrease this week. God send it."

Sure enough, as fall turned to winter and the weather became colder, the plague deaths began to subside.

At the end of the year, as people began cautiously returning to the city, John Graunt published his analysis of the epidemic. Called *London's dreadful visitation, or, A collection of all the Bills of Mortality for this present year*, it estimated that 68,000 people out of a population of 450,000 had died of plague. In a single year, the disease had wiped out 15 percent of London's population.

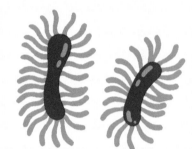

# NEW KNOWLEDGE, BUT NO CURE

By looking carefully at statistics, John Graunt helped people realize that epidemics could be predicted: high numbers of unusual deaths might point to the start of an outbreak of disease. People no longer had to look to the stars for signs of a coming epidemic; they just had to pay attention to what was happening around them. It was the beginning of a more scientific approach to disease control and prevention.

Still, much about plague remained a puzzle in 1665. How did the disease start? How did it spread? Did you catch it from breathing infected air? From contact with a victim? Could you get it from something you ate or drank? There were no answers to these questions, which made preventing and treating plague a risky guessing game.

## GRAUNT'S LEGACY

John Graunt's discovery that plague years were preceded by "sickly years" was a huge step forward in tracking diseases. His recommendation that doctors and health officials pay close attention to all unexplained increases in death rates is still helping epidemiologists pinpoint and stop disease outbreaks today.

It was only *after* the Spanish influenza pandemic in the early 20th century that investigator Wade Hampton Frost realized the rates of pneumonia had been unusually high in the months leading up to the massive outbreak of the flu in U.S. Army camps. Looking back, Wade suspected that what doctors had been calling pneumonia had really been early cases of Spanish influenza.

If someone had remembered the lesson of John Graunt and looked into the sudden jump in pneumonia cases, it might have led to an earlier identification of the illness. The Spanish flu swept through the United States before going global and killing millions worldwide in the winter of 1918.

In 2019, when doctors in Wuhan, China, noticed more pneumonia cases than usual, they were quick to let the authorities know—hoping to avert another pandemic. But the virus had a head start.

# UNEQUAL TREATMENT

In 1665, only the wealthy and middle class could afford doctors. The thousands of poor people who suffered from plague during the London epidemic mostly relied on low-cost home remedies.

A booklet from the Royal College of Physicians called *Certain Necessary Directions for the Prevention and Cure of the Plague* recommended this surefire method for treating painful swollen lymph glands, or buboes: "Pull off the feathers from the tails of living cocks, hens, pigeons, or chickens, and holding their bills, hold them hard to the Botch or Swelling and so keep them at that part until they [the birds] die; and by this means draw out the poison."

No chickens handy? There were alternatives: "Take a great onion, hollow it, put into it a fig cut small ... put it into a wet paper, and roast it in embers; apply it hot unto the tumour."

One popular remedy was called Venice Treacle (a treacle is a thick syrup). To make it, you'd need nearly 60 ingredients, from cinnamon, pepper, and cloves to exotic items like viper flesh, opium, beaver glands, and Dead Sea salts. Vipers all sold out? London Treacle was a simpler option—a mixture of cumin seeds, bayberries, snake root, cloves, and honey.

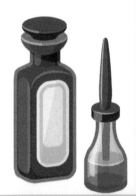

To avoid catching plague, some doctors held gold coins in their mouths while they treated patients, believing the precious metal protected them. Others recommended burning herbs and spices mixed with vinegar or tar to clean the air. So many people believed that smoking tobacco would prevent plague that schoolboys were punished if they forgot to smoke each morning before their prayers. Some people wore amulets filled with toad poison to ward off the disease. And con artists sold worthless powders and mixtures, passing them off as exotic wonder drugs: powdered unicorn horn, phoenix eggs, and the kidney stones of camels.

There was no way to cure plague, and doctors could do little to treat it. Bleeding had been recommended as a cure for fevers since ancient Greek and Roman times. Although people often died from loss of blood, doctors continued to bleed their patients. Sweating was another common treatment. It was based on the idea that because plague caused fevers, it should be treated with heat. Doctors piled on the blankets and stoked up a fire near the victim's bed, hoping that their patient would sweat out the plague poison. If neither bleeding nor sweating worked, there was opium to dull your pain (if you could afford it). When that failed, there was only prayer left.

According to John Graunt's statistics, there were only 9,967 births in London that year, compared to 97,306 burials. Some wondered if the city's population would ever recover.

John pointed out that London was an incredibly dangerous place to live at all times. Every year there were far more deaths in the city than there were births, and yet the population continued to grow because people from the surrounding countryside were constantly coming to London, looking for work and a better life. John predicted that within a few years, London's population would rebound, thanks to newcomers from the country. Again, he was right. Slowly, life began to return to normal in the city, as people forgot the year of terror and death.

# FINDING ANSWERS IN HONG KONG

More than 200 years after the epidemic in London, scientists finally identified the source of plague. In 1894, an epidemic of bubonic plague in Hong Kong killed 80,000 people. The governor, Sir William Robinson, called for scientists to come to Hong Kong to search for solutions and save the city. A famous Japanese scientist, Shibasaburo Kitasato, answered his plea.

Shibasaburo's arrival was celebrated in the papers, and he was given his own laboratory and a staff of assistants. Nobody paid much attention to another foreign researcher who answered the call for help. Alexander Yersin was a young Swiss bacteriologist—a specialist studying disease-carrying microbes, and how to cure or treat the illnesses they cause—who had been practicing medicine in the French colony of Indochina (now the countries of Vietnam and Cambodia). As an unknown scientist, Alexander didn't get the same warm welcome as the famous Shibasaburo. The Hong Kong officials didn't even offer him a laboratory. He had to pay to have his own lab built, a lowly straw hut not far from the much grander building occupied by Shibasaburo.

The two scientists were soon racing to be the first to discover the source of plague. The competition was so fierce that Shibasaburo tried to prevent Alexander from getting access to the bodies of plague victims. Alexander had to bribe the soldiers guarding the plague wards of hospitals to bring him the blood and tissue samples he needed.

That June, each man announced that he had successfully isolated the bacteria that causes plague.

# THE COTTON CONNECTION

London's great plague may have started when infected rats and their fleas hitched a ride to the city on bales of cotton imported from Holland. Just the year before, more than 50,000 people had died in a plague epidemic in Amsterdam, Holland, and there was a busy trade in cotton between the two cities. The first deaths in the London epidemic happened in a neighborhood called St. Giles in the Fields, where many dock workers lived. These workers could have been bitten by plague-infected fleas while unloading bales of cotton from the boats and bringing it into the city for sale.

Ironically, John Graunt may have been selling cloth made from that cotton in his shop, while spending his evenings tracking the spread of the epidemic it had caused through his city. Trade, travel, and disease have a long history of connection, from the trade caravans that brought plague rats to Europe from Central Asia, to the slave ships that carried mosquitoes breeding yellow fever to the United States, to today's international flights that can carry virus-infected humans anywhere they want to go. Whenever humans have found a way to make travel easier and faster, they have also made the spread of disease easier and faster.

At first, Shibasaburo was credited with the discovery, but then the scientific community decided that Alexander had been first, and the bacteria was named *Yersinia pestis* in his honor.

A few years later, French researcher Paul-Louis Simond discovered that fleas called *Xenopsylla cheopis* transferred the infection from rat to rat; when a rat died, its fleas sometimes jumped to a nearby human. Their bites passed the disease to humans. It took nearly 40 years for Simond's research to be accepted by the scientific and medical communities, but the mystery of plague was finally solved.

# THE FUTURE OF PLAGUE

Today, plague can be successfully treated with antibiotics if patients get medical attention in time. But the disease is still a feared killer. In 1993, South and Central India were rattled by a severe earthquake that damaged a number of cities, including Bangalore, Bombay, Hyderabad, and Madras, as well as many smaller villages and towns. In the earthquake's aftermath, huge shantytowns and slums sprang up to house people who had been left homeless by the disaster. The shantytowns also sheltered large numbers of rats.

In September 1994, plague broke out in one of the largest slums, in the city of Surat. Fifty-five people died—an insignificant number compared to the terrible death tolls of the medieval plague epidemics, but enough to make headlines around the world. Commercial air traffic to and from India stopped, the stock market in India crashed, trade halted, and the media went crazy speculating about the possibility that plague could spread to other countries, triggering a massive pandemic. Luckily, it didn't happen.

# A PERFECT PAIR: CITIES AND DISEASE

As soon as humans started living in permanent settlements, we opened the door to disease-causing microbes. Disease spreads easily in crowded conditions, and densely packed cities with poor sanitation are the perfect breeding ground for epidemics. Until the 20th century, so many city dwellers died each year from infectious diseases that without a steady stream of new arrivals from the countryside, most cities would have soon become ghost towns.

Plague was one of the most feared diseases because its deadly epidemics seemed to come out of nowhere. And in fact, the agent responsible for transmitting plague to humans is almost invisible. The culprit is the rat flea.

Attracted by humans' garbage, rats had moved into the settlements, bringing along their annoying roommates: *Yersinia pestis* (the bacteria that causes plague) in their guts and bloodstreams, and the fleas in their fur. Once a flea bites a rat infected with *Yersinia*, it carries the bacteria along to the next rat—or person—it dines on. In the crowded, unsanitary cities, fleas jumped easily from rat to human. For many unlucky people, those flea bites weren't only itchy—they were deadly.

As trade routes were established between cities, rats carrying plague went along for the ride. They spread across Asia and Europe, touching off the bubonic plague pandemic of the 1300s and the epidemics of plague that followed, including the Great Plague of London.

# THREE PLAGUES, ONE CAUSE

There are three types of plague: bubonic, pneumonic, and septicemic. All three forms of plague are caused by the same bacteria, *Yersinia pestis*.

Bubonic plague is the most famous and the most feared, but it is actually the least deadly of the three. In bubonic plague, the bacteria attack the lymphatic system, causing lymph nodes in the patient's neck, underarms, or groin to develop painful swellings (traditionally called buboes), as well as reddish or purple markings on the skin. In 17th-century England, these round marks were known as "plague tokens." Before the buboes or plague tokens appear, the patient suffers fever, headaches, chills, vomiting, and extreme exhaustion. More than half of all bubonic plague sufferers died within two weeks of the appearance of buboes.

Pneumonic plague is even more deadly. It attacks the lungs and spreads through the air when victims cough and sneeze. Nearly everyone infected with pneumonic plague will die within two to four days. It starts with fever and a headache, but soon the victim begins coughing up blood and their lungs fill with fluid until they can no longer breathe.

In septicemic plague, the rarest form of the disease, the bacteria infect the patient's bloodstream. Death can happen so quickly that sometimes no symptoms appear. When there are symptoms, they include fever and weakness, followed by bleeding from the mouth and nose and internal bleeding. Without treatment, victims of septicemic plague will die in less than a day.

Today, antibiotics can successfully treat about 85 percent of cases of plague—if the drugs are started during the first 24 hours after infection.

Although plague is considered a disease of the past, it is alive and well and living in rodents around the world. Plague is endemic in part of Africa, including the island of Madagascar, where the disease infects a few hundred people each year. In 2017, Madagascar had an outbreak of plague that was traced back to a man who developed symptoms while traveling across the island in a shared public taxi. Thirty-one people who came into contact with him came down with plague, and four people died. The World Health Organization considers plague a "re-emerging disease"—a possible threat that requires constant monitoring.

## ADDICTED TO STATISTICS

In 2020, the world tracked the emergence of new cases of COVID-19 day by day (and even hour by hour) in the news and on social media. In 1665, people watched the numbers published in the Bills of Mortality just as eagerly. At least 5,000 copies of the bills were printed every week, and people snatched up the latest issue to find out which neighborhoods had new cases and whether the epidemic was showing signs of slowing down.

"The Bill of Mortality, to all our griefs, is increased by 399 this week, and the increase is general through the whole city and suburbs, which makes us all sad," wrote Londoner Samuel Pepys on November 9, 1665. Anyone following the toll of COVID-19 deaths, in the news and on social media, would understand just how Pepys must have felt.

# CHAPTER 2

# PLOTTING A MYSTERY

## THE SOHO CHOLERA OUTBREAK, 1854

"Sarah, wake up. The baby's crying."

Sarah Lewis groaned and rolled over, trying to ignore her husband's whispers. It felt as if she'd only just closed her eyes. How could the baby be awake already?

She squinted at the light streaming through her thin curtains and listened to the city waking up. Here in London's crowded Soho district, in the heart of the world's biggest city, the noise never entirely went away, even at night, but it did quiet down. Now the noise was building again, as the 2 million residents of London began their day. Sarah could hear the clatter of horses' hooves, the trundle of wagons and carriages rolling over cobbled streets, the shouts of vendors and beggars and newspaper boys. Cutting through it all was the earsplitting jangle of a hopeful early-morning organ grinder.

Sarah yawned. It sounded like morning had come to Broad Street. But what had Thomas meant about the baby crying? Their daughter Frances, just six months old, was fretful and sickly, and they were used to waking up to her wails. But there were no cries this morning that Sarah could hear.

She lay still and concentrated. There was the deep, regular breathing of her husband lying beside her, and the lighter breaths of her two older children, sleeping on their pallets on the floor alongside the bed. And yes, there was a tiny whimpering, barely audible, coming from the baby's cradle.

Throwing back the sheets, Sarah rose and crossed the room to check on little Frances. She bent over the cradle, crooning a soft morning greeting, but the smile on her face quickly changed to wide-eyed alarm.

Frances was thrashing in pain. Her small, pale face glistened with sweat, and her clothes and bedding were soaked with watery diarrhea. Sarah snatched up her baby and rushed to her husband. "Thomas, run for the doctor," she implored. "Right away!"

# NOTHING TO FRET ABOUT

Dr. Rogers, when he arrived later that morning, calmed Sarah's fears. The baby was simply suffering from summer diarrhea, he explained. It wasn't unusual for young children in hot weather. However, Frances would need careful nursing to bring her back to health. He recommended giving the baby a small spoonful of castor oil or syrup of rhubarb to expel the harmful illness, and a teaspoonful of brandy mixed with hot water to calm the baby's stomach. To ease the cramps that had her daughter curled in pain, Sarah could apply a mustard plaster, made by mixing flour, water, and mustard powder, to the baby's tummy. If that didn't work, she could send to the local chemist's shop for laudanum. A few drops diluted in water would soon quiet little Frances.

"Terrible smell in the streets today, isn't there?" the doctor said, as he packed up his medical bag. "Not surprising that the child's ill, with such foul air about."

Taking him to the front door, Sarah pointed out the opening to the cesspool, a brick-lined underground pit that held the household's sewage. It was just beside the front step, and directly under the Lewis family's windows. "The smell is dreadful in this warm weather, but the cesspool's so handy for throwing out the slops. And 40 Broad Street's the best house on the street for a young family: we've got the water pump just beside us, so we can fill the water bucket on the same trip," she explained.

That afternoon, Sarah did just that. While baby Frances tossed in an uneasy doze in her cradle, her mother wrung out the dirty sheets, which had been soaking all morning in buckets of water. A full bucket in each hand, Sarah made her way carefully out the front door and down the steps, tipping the contents—the disgusting greenish soup of diarrhea and water made her stomach turn—into the cesspool. Then she continued over a few paces to join the lineup at the Broad Street water pump, refilling her buckets with wash water after a short wait.

# THE ANGEL OF DEATH VISITS

Frances's summer diarrhea was getting worse. Soon the baby was so weak she couldn't even whimper. Her eyes were sunk into her head, and her skin took on a bluish tinge. Sarah fought back her worry and kept busy nursing: gently rocking the cradle, quietly singing, stroking Frances's back. She only left the family's small room to empty the slop pail or to fetch more water.

Usually Sarah loved the chatter and gossip in the lineup at the pump. Now, with all her energies concentrated on the small, fragile life at home, she didn't linger to listen to the latest neighborhood news. Even so, she was aware that all was not right on Broad Street—a strange silence had come over the place.

Where was the clatter and turmoil, the nonstop rumble of wagons, the shouts of the street sellers? Even the organ grinders had deserted Broad Street, it seemed. The only sounds Sarah now heard from outside in the wee hours of the night were occasional running footsteps or muffled cries. That night, there was the sound of someone sobbing.

Sarah's husband, Thomas, a police constable, knew only too well what was wrong, but he didn't want to worry her. Finally, on the third evening of baby Frances's illness, he arrived home and sat down heavily at the table. "Sarah," he said flatly, "there's sickness and death all through Soho. I've seen the hearse outside almost every house up and down Broad Street. There are so many dead, they're piling them two and three deep in the undertaker's wagon. It's cholera, so they say. Everyone who can is leaving. We've got to go too. Perhaps my brother in the country will take us in."

He handed his wife a newspaper. "Look here. It's even in the papers."

Reluctantly, Sarah read the article he pointed out: ". . . this district was attacked by a pestilence which has unfortunately swept away a large number of persons who were, the day before, in perfect health. On Friday morning people might be seen before break of day running in all directions for medical advice. The angel of death had spread his wings over the place . . . it becomes the duty of all who have an interest in the welfare of the community to investigate the causes of this sudden and frightful attack."

Her face grim, Sarah thrust the paper back. "We'll keep the windows shut tight against the sickness. We won't go out unless we must. But to move that child now would be the death of her."

Sarah's voice was defiant, but she was fighting back tears. Like everyone in London, she knew that cholera was almost always fatal. The doctors suspected it came from poisoned air rising from garbage heaps, the polluted river, and the raw sewage running in the city's gutters. With the heavy summer heat hanging over London, the stink of rot and sewage was growing worse each day. But until Frances had recovered, they had to stay put and hope for the best.

# IT'S ALL GONE QUIET

The next day—September 2—Dr. Rogers returned to check on Frances. In the Lewis family's room, there was not a sound. Thomas sat at the table, his head buried in his hands. Sarah was on her knees by the tiny cradle. At the doctor's step, they turned to look at him, their faces pinched and drawn, their eyes burning. After four days of suffering, baby Frances had died. Dr. Rogers noted on the death certificate that the cause of death was "exhaustion, after an attack of diarrhea four days previous."

By now, Broad Street was almost deserted. There was no one lined up at the pump; the shops were closed; every house had its curtains pulled shut. Along the two short blocks of Broad Street stood 49 houses—formerly grand houses of the aristocracy, now mostly

# CURES FOR A PENNY

Cholera was one of the most feared diseases of the 19th century. It could kill healthy people in a matter of hours. People were prepared to try anything to keep it away, and newspapers were full of advertisements for miraculous remedies, like "SAUNDER'S ANTI-MEPHITIC FLUID. This powerful disinfectant destroys foul smells in a moment and impregnates the air with a refreshing fragrance."

Doctors fought cholera with laudanum, calomel, and camphor. Laudanum, similar to today's morphine, took away patients' pain, but it was highly addictive, and both children and adults could easily overdose on it. In small doses, calomel caused vomiting and diarrhea, and in large doses it gave the patient mercury poisoning. Camphor, a strong-smelling oil from the wood of the camphor laurel tree, is also poisonous.

As it turns out, the cure for cholera couldn't be simpler: clean water, and lots of it. Cholera causes massive fluid loss from vomiting and diarrhea, but if patients can stay hydrated, they nearly always survive. Today, cholera patients take oral rehydration salts or receive fluids intravenously. If properly treated, less than 1 percent of people with cholera will die.

rented out to poor laborers—that offered shelter to an astounding 860 people. Almost every room housed an entire family, who did their cooking, washing, sleeping, and living within its crowded space. Squeezed in behind the houses and along the alleys were cowsheds, slaughterhouses, and breweries, even a factory for making bullets. All had now gone quiet.

On September 3, the silence on Broad Street was broken by distant footsteps, coming closer. A man appeared. He headed straight for the street's water pump. From a leather case, he took out a small glass bottle, which he filled with water. He capped it, put it to his eye, and stared at the clear liquid for a moment or two, then put the bottle back into the case and strapped it closed. From the clinking as he walked off, it seemed that there might be other bottles inside as well.

This unusual man was a doctor and a scientist, and at a time when most people broke down in panic at the words "cholera epidemic," to him the Broad Street outbreak was a golden opportunity. He was John Snow—a man who thought he had solved the mystery of cholera, and who was looking for a way to prove it.

## KNOW YOUR ENEMY

Dr. John Snow had been studying cholera for more than 20 years. When he was still training to become a doctor, John had been sent to the town of Killingworth in northern England to help miners who were dying from a cholera epidemic. He was appalled by the terrible conditions in the mines, and he suspected that they were linked to the disease outbreak.

In a letter to his family, he wrote, "The pit is one huge privy, and of course the men always take their victuals with unwashed hands." We now know that cholera is spread when infected fecal matter gets into food or water, but at the time no one understood this.

The accepted explanation was that cholera was caused by "miasma," a fog of infected air rising from piles of garbage and sewage. John disagreed. How could bad air cause the severe diarrhea he'd seen among the cholera-stricken miners? Since the disease affected the digestive system, he suspected that cholera was caused by something you ingested—something in food or water.

At first, John kept his suspicions to himself—after all, he hadn't even finished medical school yet. He knew his ideas would be laughed at. But he didn't forget about them—he waited for an opportunity to prove his theory.

By the 1840s, Dr. John Snow had a thriving medical practice as one of the world's first anesthesiologists (pronounced an-es-thee-zee-awl-o-jists)—a specialist who gives patients medication so they don't feel pain during surgery. "Sleeping gases" (chloroform and ether) had been discovered that, when inhaled, made people temporarily unconscious. This was a breakthrough for surgeons (and patients!). Before the discovery of ether, surgeons had to operate on people who were fully awake. It was so terribly painful, sometimes patients would leap off the operating table in the middle of surgery and try to escape.

John invented a regulator to deliver a safe, steady flow of gas to patients. He became so famous for his skill that he was asked to give chloroform to Queen Victoria during the births of two of her children.

John's growing knowledge about the properties of gases made him even more convinced that miasma couldn't be the cause of cholera. He'd learned how concentrated the doses of chloroform and ether had to be in order to put patients to sleep even briefly, so it didn't make sense that clouds of bad air could infect people throughout an entire city. And if bad air was really causing cholera, why didn't everyone develop the disease? The theory of miasma seemed full of logical inconsistencies, but he had no way to test his suspicions.

Then cholera came back. A new epidemic of the disease was sweeping Europe, and in the spring of 1853, a year before the Broad Street outbreak, the disease hit South London, the part of the city that lay along the south bank of the River Thames.

Still no one understood what caused cholera, or how it spread. Theories abounded. Some speculated that the people in the poor neighborhoods along the river were "morally suscep- tible"—defects in their character made them prone to developing cholera. The "miasmatists" insisted that it was the smell from the neighborhoods and the river that caused the disease.

John Snow started wondering where the people along the river got their drinking water.

# THE GRAND EXPERIMENT

There was only one way to find out—by asking. So that summer, on his own, in his evenings and on weekends, John Snow went from house to house in South London, knocking on doors, inquiring how many people in each home had gotten sick and how many had died. Then he would follow up with an unexpected question: "Do you know which company supplies your water?"

In the neighborhoods south of the river, most people no longer got their water from public pumps, but had it piped in from the River Thames. There were two private water companies supplying that part of London: Lambeth and Southwark & Vauxhall. While Lambeth piped in water from a relatively clean part of the river upstream, Southwark & Vauxhall drew their water downstream from the main sewer lines,

# THE GREAT DEBATE:
# MIASMA VS. GERMS

Today, it seems odd that so many people, including most doctors, believed disease floated around us in invisible clouds called miasma. How did this idea get started, and why did people believe in it for so long?

The term "miasma" comes from the ancient Greek word for pollution. Miasma was thought to be a poisonous mist or vapor, rising up from rotting garbage and organic matter. Even the word "malaria," for instance, comes from the Italian *mal aria*: literally, "bad air." By the 19th century, nearly everyone equated bad smells with disease.

Even after scientists like John Snow—and later Robert Koch, who in the 1880s was the first to identify the bacteria that causes cholera—proved that germs, not miasma, were the sources of disease, many people refused to change their opinions. Florence Nightingale, the founder of modern nursing, believed until the day she died in 1910 that miasma was the source of many diseases, and she championed cleanliness, hygiene, fresh air, and sunshine as ways to prevent and cure disease. Nightingale's emphasis on the importance of high standards of hygiene in hospitals has saved millions of lives, and she was right that there is a connection between poor sanitation and diseases such as cholera and typhoid. But the connection is germs, not smells.

which poured the city's waste into the water. Would that difference affect who got sick? John Snow suspected it would.

Significantly, there was no predictable pattern to the water supply system: one house might be supplied by Lambeth, while all its nearest neighbors got water from Southwark & Vauxhall. If John could show that cholera struck only the homes supplied with dirty water, it would be strong proof that miasma was not the cause. He hoped that his "Grand Experiment" would establish once and for all that cholera was spread through contaminated water.

Before John could complete his investigations, the Broad Street outbreak began. Could he apply the techniques he had been using in South London, find the source of the outbreak, and do it fast enough to halt the epidemic, or to stop it from spreading beyond Soho? He knew he had to try.

# THE SEARCH BROADENS

John marched up and down the streets of Soho, taking samples from all the local pumps. He hoped he'd be able to identify some contaminant. But when he got the vials of water home, they all seemed to be clear.

John wasn't easily discouraged. He took to the streets again, knocking on doors, asking the same odd questions: "Has anyone in this house had cholera? Where do you get your water?" Over and over, he heard the same answer: "The Broad Street pump."

There were a few places that had escaped the epidemic, but even these exceptions seemed to point back to the pump. Just around the corner from Broad Street, at 50 Poland Street, there had been only two deaths reported at the St. James Workhouse, a charity home for more than 500 of Soho's poorest men, women, and children. Why had the cholera hardly touched these residents, while killing so many of their neighbors? The answer was that the workhouse had its own well, right on the premises.

The other location in the neighborhood that seemed to have been passed over by the epidemic was a brewery on Broad Street. When John Snow asked the brewery owner where his workers got their water, he learned they were given a ration of beer every day and drank that instead.

By now, John was convinced that the Broad Street pump was the source of the outbreak. But there was one death he couldn't account for. Susannah Eley, an elderly woman living across town in the Hampstead Heath neighborhood, had died of cholera on September 2. The date put her right in the midst of the Broad Street outbreak, yet what could her connection to the Soho epidemic be?

With a few more questions up and down Broad Street, John got his answer.

Susannah's sons operated the Eley Percussion Cap factory on Broad Street. Every day, they sent their mother a jug of cold water, fresh from the Broad Street pump, because she insisted that Broad Street had the best-tasting water in all of London. Susannah Eley's love for the water from the Broad Street pump had been fatal.

# CAN YOU "HANDLE" THE TRUTH?

By Thursday, September 7, more than 500 people had died in an area of only a few blocks. An emergency meeting of the parish council was called. Worried men in tall hats and dark suits gathered in the parish hall to see what could be done to halt the deaths and suffering.

Just as they were agreeing that burning sulfur in the streets to disinfect the air was the best strategy, a stranger, sitting alone in the back of the hall, asked permission to speak. The council members listened in astonishment as Dr. John Snow laid out the results of his door-to-door research. The council was skeptical about John's outlandish water theory. However, they reasoned that preventing people from drinking the Broad Street water could do no harm, and it just might do some good.

The next day, workmen were sent out with instructions to remove the handle of the Broad Street pump. The spread of cholera, which had already been declining in the neighborhood, stopped altogether. The epidemic was over.

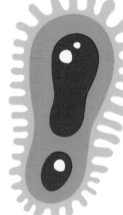

But the Soho Parish Council and the London Board of Health were not convinced that contaminated water had caused the outbreak or that the well was a source of contamination. They asked John Snow to continue his investigation and report back to them.

One man from the council volunteered to assist John with his investigation. But he wasn't an ally—at least, not at first. Henry Whitehead was the new assistant minister at St. Luke's, the local church, and he was convinced that John's theory was just plain wrong.

## THE PICTURE COMES INTO FOCUS

Despite their differences, the shy doctor and the young minister made a good team. Henry Whitehead was just 29 years old, and St. Luke's was his first parish. He was full of energy, and he already knew many of the residents of Soho by name. Day after day he paced the streets, knocking on doors, trying to track down residents who had fled the neighborhood in the early days of the outbreak. He visited some homes four or five times, until he was satisfied that he'd gathered all the information he could.

While Henry walked the streets, John spent hours every night in his study, poring over the data they'd collected. Frustratingly, there seemed little left to learn. Then one night, John tried something new. He took his list of confirmed cases of cholera and transferred the information onto a map of the neighborhood. He drew a black bar for every case reported from each address. Soon there were clusters of black bars up and down the winding streets. He studied the map. Something was missing.

John picked up his pen and marked in the locations of all the water pumps in the neighborhood.

By the time he put his pen down, he saw that he had drawn a picture of the epidemic. The black bars radiated out from the Broad Street pump, thickest near the pump and getting less frequent farther away. He felt certain the map would make an impression on the council in a way his earlier lists and tables hadn't been able to. But he still faced a problem. Could this map convince Henry Whitehead?

# THE FINAL CLUE

We'll never know whether John's map alone would have been enough to convince Henry Whitehead and the parish council. Because at almost the same time, Henry Whitehead uncovered the last piece of the Broad Street puzzle. One evening, sifting through the piles of documents that filled his study, his eyes landed on a single line that had until then escaped his notice: "Death from exhaustion, after an attack of diarrhea four days previous." It was little Frances Lewis's death certificate.

Until now, Frances's death hadn't been considered part of the cholera outbreak, but Henry realized that she might have been one of its many victims. He was surprised that a young baby had withstood the illness for four days, when adults often died of the disease in a matter of hours. Four days. That meant Frances had taken ill before any other cases were reported. He looked again at the death certificate to be sure, and noticed the address: 40 Broad Street, right next door to the Broad Street pump.

Henry's hands, holding the death certificate, began trembling. His brain whirled, at last making the connections that had eluded him and John Snow. Here was evidence of a case of cholera that had started *two days before* the general outbreak in the neighborhood, and it was very likely that the victim's diarrhea had been disposed of near the Broad Street pump, which was the connection between all the other cases in the epidemic. Had Frances's cholera-laden diarrhea contaminated the water of the Broad Street pump, and led to the outbreak? Henry got up. Despite the late hour, he knew John Snow would want to hear about his discovery.

The next day, Sarah Lewis answered a knock to find two serious-looking gentlemen on her doorstep. They'd come, they explained, to ask about her baby's illness. When had Frances first gotten sick? Where did the family get their water? Where did their waste go?

Sarah showed them the cesspool opening at the foot of the stairs, where several times a day she had poured out the water she'd used for soaking the dirty sheets and diapers. Seeing that the cesspool was just steps away from the Broad Street pump, John and Henry knew they had found the source of the epidemic.

# TOOL OF THE TRADE: MAPPING OUTBREAKS

John Snow's map of the Soho cholera outbreak is still studied by students of epidemiology. John was the first to use maps to show how disease outbreaks are linked to risk factors in the environment. In the Soho epidemic, when the city officials saw how the cases clustered around the location of the pump, they realized that closing the pump could stop the outbreak.

Today, epidemiologists map outbreaks using sophisticated software that allows them to track and predict the spread of epidemics through both space and time. Mapping disease outbreaks is more complicated now than it was for John Snow because of the way that travel has changed. In the 1800s, travel was slow. Maps of disease outbreaks tended to show ripples radiating out from a single point, like the waves spreading from a stone dropped in a pond.

Air travel changed that pattern completely. Now, maps of disease outbreaks show clusters appearing randomly across the globe—Shanghai, Brussels, Vancouver, Mexico City—and they look more like bursts of fireworks than ripples in a pond. But researchers have realized there is a pattern to what looks like chaos. International travel today happens through a linked network of airports. Substitute the typical map of the world with a map that shows the flights between different cities, and the randomness of the outbreaks becomes more predictable, resolving into the same outward ripples as John Snow's original map.

# THE DIRTY TRUTH

John and Henry made such a convincing case that the parish council ordered the cesspool in front of 40 Broad Street and the well under the corner pump to be dug up. The engineers called in for the job found that the brick lining of the cesspool had decayed, and the earth between the cesspool and the well was soaked with sewage. Anything going into the cesspool would find its way—and fast—into the water in the well. The cholera from Frances Lewis's diarrhea had traveled into the street's drinking water, setting off the cholera epidemic.

A few years after John Snow's investigation, the city of London installed the modern world's first major sewer system. Led by

# DO YOU SMELL WHAT I SMELL?

In 1854, London was the biggest city to date in the history of humankind, with a population of 2.5 million people and growing. But it didn't have a citywide sewer system, a city dump, or even one city garbage collector. The result? London was drowning in its own filth.

Many houses weren't connected to a sewer and relied instead on cesspools, large underground pits where each household deposited its waste. When the pit filled up, the landlord called in the "night-soil men," who came and emptied it, hauling the contents away to the edge of town. This system had worked well for a long time, but London was growing fast, and the edge of town was getting farther and farther away. The night-soil men raised their prices, and soon landlords were putting off having their cesspools emptied. The cesspools frequently overflowed, flooding cellars with human waste.

The situation wasn't much better for those who lived in houses connected to sewers and with running water. The sewers emptied straight into the Thames, the river that flowed through the heart of London. And where did the city's drinking water supplies come from? Why, from the Thames!

Using the river as both a sewer and a water source created a perfect environment for spreading disease. All that sewage also made the city incredibly smelly. And human waste wasn't the only problem. London was full of industry: breweries and tanneries, forges and factories. And full of animals: horses, chickens, pigs, and cows were kept in small enclosures. They all added to the waste and garbage and smells. So it's not too surprising that people connected the epidemics that regularly raged across the city with London's most immediately identifiable problem: its stink.

engineer Joseph Bazalgette, the city built 132 km (82 mi) of brick-lined sewers to sweep London's waste far down the Thames. It was one of the biggest civil engineering projects ever undertaken, and it made London the most modern city of the time. Cities throughout Europe and North America were soon following London's lead by building sewer systems to safeguard the health of their inhabitants.

# CHOLERA: EVERYTHING OLD IS NEW AGAIN

Think cholera outbreaks are ancient history? Think again.

Between 1816 and 1923, cholera killed over 2 million people worldwide. The disease came in waves of pandemics, with just a few years of calm in between. Then, for over 40 years in the middle of the 20th century, cholera seemed to vanish. There's a fairly simple explanation: modern sanitation. As modern sewer systems and water treatment became the norm across the developed world, cholera had far fewer opportunities to spread. From being the scourge of cities, it went to being an almost unknown disease in North America, Europe, and Australia. But for the more than 2 billion people in the world who still lack access to clean water, the threat of cholera never went away.

Cholera gets a foothold when natural disasters strike, or when war or instability pushes large numbers of people into crammed refugee camps. Wherever there are crowded living conditions, a lack of clean water and sewage disposal, and too few doctors, drugs, and hospitals, cholera has a chance to thrive.

That was the situation in Haiti after a massive earthquake struck the island in 2010, making a million people homeless. The United Nations sent forces to the island to help in the aftermath of the quake, including some peacekeepers from Nepal who became sick with cholera.

Water and sanitation systems had been damaged in the earthquake and the disease spread quickly. Then in 2016, Hurricane Matthew hit the island, causing more destruction, and the disease surged back.

When the epidemic finally ended in 2019, more than 600,000 people had been infected and almost 10,000 had died. Epidemiologists in Haiti continue monitoring and testing, ready to act fast if cholera comes back.

# CHAPTER 3

# DID THE MOSQUITO DO IT?

## YELLOW FEVER IN CUBA, 1900

"You know, James, I've never thought of myself as sentimental, but I can't help feeling sorry for these poor creatures we're experimenting on. Take this old lady, for example. She's spent her whole life in captivity, she hasn't had a good meal in days—no wonder she's so weak and listless!"

As he spoke, Dr. Jesse Lazear lifted a test tube up to the light and tapped it gently, dislodging the mosquito inside from her perch on the side of the tube. Briefly, the insect lifted into the air, but she soon settled back down to cling to the slippery glass walls of her prison, her wings drooping.

"You're right, Jesse," observed his lab companion, Dr. James Carroll. "That little skeeter looks like she's on her last legs. Not much pep left in her, is there?"

Dr. Jesse Lazear smiled grimly. "She's not going to live out the day, in my opinion. Unless, that is, somebody can tempt her to feed on them. She bit a fever patient 12 days ago, and she's had nothing since then. She couldn't muster the energy to bite this morning's volunteer. I need another willing victim."

The two men looked at each other across the battered wooden lab table. In the silence, even the trapped mosquito seemed to be waiting to hear what would happen next.

James cleared his throat. "She'll die today unless she feeds, you say?" he asked.

"Yes, and she's almost the last hatched from that batch of eggs Dr. Finlay gave us. When they're gone, I'll have to find more eggs and raise the insects from larvae again—and it's such a chore! But the worst of it is that it will set our experiments back by days, waiting for new mosquitoes to reach maturity."

James took a deep breath and started rolling up his shirtsleeve. "Bring that test tube over here, and we'll see if her ladyship likes the taste of me."

When his friend hesitated, James laughed. "Come on, Jesse. You know as well as I do that yellow fever isn't transmitted by mosquitoes. That little imp is going to do nothing more than give me an itchy lump for a day or two. Then we'll be able to stop these foolish experiments and get back to the real work—finding the bacteria that causes the disease."

Reluctantly, Jesse Lazear picked up the test tube, pulled out the stopper, and jammed the mouth of the tube against his friend's bare arm. The mosquito fluttered aimlessly up and down, then came to rest again on the side of the test tube.

Jesse rolled his eyes, sighing in exasperation. "Just like this morning. Too weak to feed." He started to withdraw the test tube from James's arm.

"Be patient, man! Give the lady a chance to make up her mind. Maybe she's picking out the tastiest spot."

After several minutes more of waiting and watching, Jesse gave up, leaving the test tube and its indecisive inhabitant to the care of James. James sat patiently holding the tube to his forearm, silently willing the mosquito to lift up from her perch. Finally, he announced, "Success! She's done it, Jesse, she's done it!"

And that was the end of it. A few minutes out of a busy afternoon's work to make sure that an experiment stayed on schedule. James had soon put the whole thing out of his mind. The bite didn't even itch.

# THE CUBAN EXPERIMENTS

Jesse Lazear and James Carroll hadn't come to Cuba just to raise mosquitoes. Their assignment was much bigger: find the cause of yellow fever, one of the most feared and deadly diseases of the century.

As their ship sailed into the great harbor of Havana, the capital city of Cuba, both Jesse and James had been out on deck, eager to get their first sight of the famously beautiful island. Above the city rose green hills covered with waving palm and coconut trees, while the harbor was guarded by immense stone fortifications. Inside the city walls, they could glimpse gaily painted homes, the tall spires of churches, and the elaborately decorated buildings that had given the city the name *Ciudad des las Columnas* (City of the Columns). In the middle of the harbor, rising up out of the water, was the black hulk of a destroyed ship.

It was the wreck of the *Maine*, a U.S. Army ship that had been blown up by the Spanish two years earlier, killing more than 260 sailors on board and setting off the bitterly fought Spanish-American War. The two doctors had often heard the rallying cry echo through the United States: "Remember the *Maine*! To hell with Spain!" Now here it was before them, the ruined ship that had put their country on the path to war—a conflict that had resulted in the victorious U.S. taking control of the Spanish island of Cuba.

In 1900, there were more than 50,000 American soldiers occupying Cuba, and the army was worried. The war might be over, but their troops were still dying—of yellow fever. In fact, already more soldiers had been lost to yellow fever than had been killed in the fighting. And with ships full of soldiers coming and going constantly between the island and the nearby American mainland, the risk of a sick soldier setting off an epidemic in an American city was growing by the day.

It was a risk the U.S. Army was determined to put a stop to. Terrible epidemics of yellow fever had ravaged cities across the United States all through the 18th and 19th centuries, with the sickness becoming known and feared as the "yellow death." During a single epidemic in Philadelphia, in 1793, 10 percent of the city's population had died. New Orleans was even more unlucky. That city had suffered six major epidemics by 1878, when it was hit again, along with 131 other cities and towns in the U.S. Nowhere, it seemed, was safe from the menace of the yellow death. But in Cuba, the U.S. Army was seizing the chance to solve the mystery of yellow fever, once and for all.

# THE FEVER FIGHTERS

Along with James Carroll and Jesse Lazear, the U.S. Army had sent two other doctors to Cuba: Major Walter Reed would lead the team, and Aristides Agramonte would assist him.

Walter and James were bacteriologists: specialists in uncovering the causes of disease and developing cures or treatments. Jesse Lazear was the head of a clinical labora- tory at Johns Hopkins University in Baltimore, and Aristides Agramonte was an experienced medical investigator. At Camp Columbia, the U.S. Army's main base in Cuba, the team's mission was simple: find the cause of yellow fever.

Simple, but incredibly risky. By agreeing to the assign- ment, each of the men knew he was putting himself at risk. Year after year, yellow fever took a terrible toll on the people of Cuba, killing hundreds or even thousands.

It started with chills and fever, a crushing headache, and aching pains in the legs and back. After three or four days, many patients recovered. But in some cases, the fever progressed to a second stage, increasing until the victim's temperature reached 40 degrees Celsius (104 degrees Fahrenheit) or more. Then the skin and the whites of the eyes began to turn yellow, or jaundiced, as the disease attacked the liver—this frightening symptom gave yellow fever its name. Next, the victims would begin to vomit black, clotted blood. Within two weeks, half of the patients who developed the second stage of the fever died.

Yellow fever snuck up on its victims mysteriously. Did you get it from contact with infected clothes or bedding? Did yellow fever germs travel from person to person through the air? Could it be transmitted through contaminated water or food? Every doctor and scientist studying the disease had a favorite theory, and there was very little hard evidence for or against any of them. That's why Walter Reed was determined that his team would follow the strictest standards of scientific inquiry. Their experiments had to be foolproof, and the results had to stand the test of time. There had been other investigations into the causes of the "yellow death," but Walter and his fellow doctors wanted theirs to be the last.

# HOME AT CAMP COLUMBIA

In late June 1900, on the spacious veranda of their new quarters at Columbia Barracks Hospital, the team met to plan their strategy. The summer rains were beginning, and they knew it meant that soon the hospital beds would fill with yellow fever patients. The doctors decided to test three theories about how the disease spread.

At the time, many people believed that yellow fever could be transmitted through contact with infected clothing and bedding. The team agreed to design experiments that would expose people to clothes that had been worn by yellow fever patients, to test this theory.

An Italian researcher, Dr. Giuseppe Sanarelli, claimed to have found a bacteria that caused yellow fever: *Bacillus icteroides*. To test these claims, the team planned to perform autopsies on yellow fever victims, remove tissue samples, and try to grow the bacteria from the samples. James Carroll's skill as a bacteriologist would be essential to these experiments.

For their third set of experiments, they decided to investigate a little-known theory from a Cuban doctor. For over 20 years, Dr. Carlos Finlay had been trying to prove that mosquitoes spread yellow fever in humans. Most people considered this a far-fetched idea, but Walter and his fellow disease detectives were determined to follow every lead. They would test Dr. Finlay's theory as well.

## FIGHTING FEVER

Before people understood that mosquitoes spread yellow fever, stopping an epidemic was almost impossible. In 1793, when yellow fever broke out in Philadelphia, doctors gave the best advice they had:

"Avoid fatigue of body and mind. Don't stand or sit in a draft, in the sun, or in the evening air."

"Dress according to the weather. Avoid intemperance. Drink sparingly of wine, beer, or cider."

"When visiting the sick, use vinegar or camphor on your handkerchief; carry it in smelling bottles; use it frequently."

"Place your patients in the center of your biggest, airiest room in beds without curtains."

"Burn gunpowder. It clears the air."

None of it worked. The epidemic killed 5,000 people in just three months, stopping only when a fall cold snap froze the mosquito larvae breeding in puddles and swamps around the city.

# INTO HAVANA

To learn more about Dr. Finlay's yellow fever mosquito experiments, Walter Reed's team set off to visit him in Havana. As their horse-drawn carriage jolted along rutted dirt roads into the city, it seemed unlikely that groundbreaking scientific research could be happening in a sleepy backwater like Cuba. But while they had little faith in the Cuban doctor's theories, they were determined to explore every possibility.

White-bearded, bespectacled Dr. Finlay welcomed them graciously, but there wasn't much small talk among the five medical men that night. Carlos Finlay got right to the point, describing his efforts to prove that mosquitoes spread yellow fever.

He'd conducted no less than 103 experiments, exposing human volunteers to the bites of mosquitoes to see if they developed the disease. But his results were ignored because he hadn't kept his volunteers in isolation. Scientists pointed out that they could just as easily have picked up yellow fever from another person as from the mosquito bite.

Carlos begged Walter and the others to complete his work. He explained that when a mosquito "bites" a person, it pierces their skin with its proboscis, or long thin nose, to suck up blood—and when the mosquito's victim is a yellow fever patient, their blood is infected with the microbes that cause the disease. Then, when the mosquito bites someone else, it transmits those microbes, causing yellow fever.

As the team left, Carlos pressed a small bowl into Jesse Lazear's hands. "Mosquito eggs," he explained. "In two weeks, you'll have a lovely batch of insects to work with. Good luck."

Back in their barracks that night, the four Americans lay awake for hours replaying Carlos's arguments in their minds. Were mosquitoes the answer to the yellow fever mystery after all? The next morning, they agreed: they would start testing the mosquito theory immediately.

Right away, they ran into a problem. In order to test Dr. Finlay's theory that mosquitoes spread yellow fever, they would need to have mosquitoes bite patients suffering from yellow fever, and then bite healthy people. If the theory was correct, their healthy test subjects would develop yellow fever. People could die from the experiments.

The doctors agreed that they could not ask the soldiers at Camp Columbia or Cubans in the surrounding area to take such a risk, unless they were also prepared to put their own lives on the line. Three weeks later, on August 27, Jesse Lazear put the mosquito on his friend James Carroll's arm.

# TROUBLES ACCUMULATE

For three days, James showed no effects from his mosquito bite. He carried on as usual, examining tissue samples under the microscope, looking for evidence of Dr. Sanarelli's *Bacillus icteroides* in yellow fever patients. Of all the team members, James was the least convinced by the mosquito transmission theory. He was sure the answer to the yellow fever mystery would be found under the microscope, not by breeding insects.

But on August 30, James began feeling feverish. He and Jesse went for a swim that afternoon to cool off, and when James emerged from the water, he started shaking, and soon he developed a blinding headache. Another army doctor looked him over and told him bluntly that he had yellow fever. James didn't believe him, and he carried on working. Yet by the next afternoon, James was lying in the yellow fever ward in Camp Columbia's hospital with a temperature of 39 degrees Celsius (102 degrees Fahrenheit), and there was no longer any question about what was making him so ill.

The research team was in shock and unsure what to do next. Walter Reed had just returned to the United States to complete a research report on an earlier study he had been involved in. Jesse and Aristides sent him a cable, letting him know about James. Overcome with guilt, Walter wrote to a friend, "I cannot begin to describe my mental distress and depression over this most unfortunate turn of affairs. We had all determined to experiment on ourselves & I should have taken the same dose had I been there. Can it be that this was the source of his infection?"

Fortunately, James's case of yellow fever wasn't fatal. Soon he was well enough to read a congratulatory letter from Walter: "Hip! Hip!

Hoorah! God be praised for the news from Cuba today—Really, I can never recall such a sense of relief in all my life, as the news of your recovery gives me! . . . God bless you, my boy." On the back of the envelope, Walter had scribbled the question that was now foremost in all of their minds: "Did the mosquito do it?"

The evidence seemed to point to the mosquito, but the scientists weren't quite convinced. James could have been infected through his exposure to yellow fever patients in the hospital, or through his work with infected tissue samples in the laboratory. The research team needed more evidence: they needed to see if a mosquito could cause yellow fever in another volunteer.

But who would volunteer for such a hazardous duty?

The solution, as it turned out, stopped by their laboratory later that day.

Private William Dean was new to Camp Columbia, and to Cuba. He'd never been exposed to any yellow fever patients, and he was curious about the unusual experiments he'd heard were going on in the ramshackle laboratory. When William passed the door to the lab that day, he glanced in and happened to meet Jesse's eye.

"You still fooling with mosquitoes, Doctor?" William asked.

"Yes," said Jesse. "Will you take a bite?"

"Sure, I ain't scared of 'em."

A week later, Aristides burst into the lab with the news that Private Dean had been admitted that morning to the camp hospital with fever, chills, and a headache—the classic early symptoms of yellow fever. Could this be the evidence they needed?

# HUMAN GUINEA PIGS

Private William Dean had a mild case of yellow fever, and he was soon on the road to recovery. With James Carroll also slowly recovering, and the evidence against the mosquitoes mounting, everything seemed to be going well for the research team. Then disaster struck.

Jesse Lazear came down with yellow fever.

How had it happened? Jesse insisted it was accidental—he had been holding a test tube against a patient when a wild mosquito landed on his hand. Rather than risk letting the mosquito in the test tube escape, Jesse had allowed the wild mosquito to bite him, confident that he was immune to yellow fever. That's what he told his colleagues, as he lay in his bed in one of the hospital's fever wards.

But later, as they were going through their research notes, James and Aristides came across a puzzling entry in Jesse's handwriting: "Sep 13: This guinea pig bitten today by a mosquito which developed from egg laid by a mosquito which bit Tanner Aug 6. This mosquito bit Suarez Aug 30, Hernandez Sep 2, De Long Sep 7, Fernandez Sep 10."

Who was the guinea pig? Could the note mean that Jesse had decided to experiment on himself, allowing mosquitoes to bite him after feeding on fever patients? Before they could confront him with their suspicions, however, Dr. Jesse Lazear died of yellow fever, just 10 days after being bitten.

## THAT BITES!

As anyone who's ever spent a hot summer night in a cottage, cabin, or tent can tell you, nothing keeps you awake at night like a mosquito buzzing in your ear. And the next day—boy, those bites really itch!

Usually, the urge to scratch for a few days is our only lasting reminder of an unpleasant encounter with a mosquito. But if you're not so lucky, the effects of a mosquito bite can be worse than an itchy lump. Much worse.

In addition to yellow fever, mosquitoes spread a number of dangerous, even deadly diseases among humans. Depending on where you live, these include malaria, dengue fever, Rift Valley fever, West Nile virus, and encephalitis. It is estimated that mosquitoes transmit these diseases to an astounding 700 million people every year.

# REED RETURNS

Walter Reed raced back to Cuba, only to find his research team in chaos. Jesse was dead, James was still very weak from his bout of yellow fever, and Aristides was deeply upset by what had befallen his colleagues. Yet, despite all the suffering, important scientific work had been done—possibly enough to establish how yellow fever was transmitted.

Walter got right to work by interviewing William Dean. To prove that the mosquito bite had led to William's illness, it was important to demonstrate that the bite was his only exposure to the disease. William insisted that he hadn't left Camp Columbia and that he hadn't been in the hospital's fever wards. It looked like an open-and-shut case.

A month later, on October 23, Walter Reed delivered a report to the American Public Health Association, describing his team's experiments in Cuba and their conclusion: "The mosquito serves as the intermediate host [the carrier] for yellow fever." The medical community was unconvinced. A single case wasn't enough to prove anything, they told Walter. He needed to test and retest, and his experiments needed to be more carefully controlled so that it was clear his research subjects were exposed to yellow fever only through the mosquito bite.

The scientists who listened to Walter's report had been respectful, but not everyone took his theory seriously. An article in the *Washington Post* called the mosquito theory "silly and nonsensical rigamarole." The ridicule only made Walter more determined. He boarded his ship back to Cuba swearing that he wouldn't leave again until he'd proven beyond a shadow of a doubt that mosquitoes spread yellow fever.

# "$100 IN AMERICAN GOLD"

Back at Camp Columbia, Walter convinced the governor-general of Cuba to give his team $10,000 to fund their experiments—the equivalent of nearly a quarter of a million dollars today. They used it to build special cabins away from the rest of the camp to keep their research subjects isolated during experiments. The new research area was called Camp Lazear, in honor of Jesse Lazear's sacrifice. But the research team still hadn't decided one thing: Who would participate in the experiments?

The three remaining doctors talked it through again and again. Despite the dangers, it still seemed as if the only way to solve the mystery was to use human volunteers. This time around, though, they would make sure that everyone who volunteered was aware that they were

# TOOL OF THE TRADE:
# HUMAN EXPERIMENTS

Walter Reed knew that to test the theory that mosquitoes transmit yellow fever, he would have to experiment on humans and that some of them might die. He wanted every volunteer to understand the risks. The forms he asked all the volunteer subjects to sign are among the earliest examples of "informed consent."

Not all experiments on humans have been as ethical. During World War II, the Nazis subjected prisoners to cruel experiments. To prevent it from happening in the future, an international agreement called the Nuremberg Code was developed. Under the code, researchers must have the consent of their research subjects, and experiments must be well-designed and safe.

Even then, researchers experimenting on humans didn't always follow the rules. In one study in the United States, Black American farmworkers who were suffering from syphilis were told that they would get free medical treatment. Instead, researchers from the U.S. Public Health Service observed them as they got sicker and sicker, in order to learn more about the disease.

The World Medical Association now requires studies with human subjects to meet high standards of ethical practice. Ethics committees at universities and research institutions review research plans before approving funding, and the principle of informed consent that Walter Reed pioneered in Cuba is central to the design of experiments with human participants.

risking their lives. They decided to only accept participants who were young (because yellow fever was more dangerous in older people), healthy, and single (so that the experiments would not end with widows or orphaned children).

Men who agreed to participate in the experiments would earn $100 in gold—that's the equivalent of more than $3,000 today. If they got sick with yellow fever, they would get another $100. For the U.S. soldiers and for the poor Cubans and Spanish immigrants in the area, that was a very tempting offer. Soon, the research team had a lineup of willing volunteers.

By the end of November, Camp Lazear was ready for its guests. The camp was really just a patch of land outside Camp Columbia, with tents for the researchers and two wooden cabins where the test subjects would stay during the experiments. Barbed-wire fences kept visitors away from the quarantine zone.

First, the researchers tested whether yellow fever could be transmitted through clothing, as many people believed. Three volunteers put on the filthy nightclothes and underwear that had been worn by yellow fever patients, and they slept in beds covered with sheets and blankets from the fever hospital. Neither the clothing nor the sheets had been washed—they were still covered with urine, feces, vomit, and blood from the terribly sick people who had used them last. For three weeks, the men stayed in the cabin. At the end of that time, no one had developed yellow fever.

They repeated the experiment three times with different volunteers. Each time, the men emerged from their ordeal free from yellow fever. The team had proven that one of the most widespread beliefs about yellow fever was wrong.

For their next experiment, they had built a cabin with a fine wire mesh screen running down the middle, splitting the interior into two isolated halves. On December 21, the researchers released 15 mosquitoes that had previously bitten fever patients into one half of the cabin. A volunteer was admitted into the midst of the buzzing insects. At the same time, by a separate door, two other volunteers entered the adjoining section of the cabin—the mosquito-free zone. The three men stayed in the cabin, together yet separated, for two days. The unlucky man in the mosquito zone was bitten again and again.

After two days, the bitten man returned to his tent while the two other volunteers stayed on in the cabin. The doctors closely monitored the bitten volunteer. On Christmas day, Walter Reed stopped by the man's tent to check on him. The volunteer, Private John Moran, was lying in bed, his face flushed, his temperature a scorching 39 degrees Celsius (102 degrees Fahrenheit). He had yellow fever.

The two volunteers in the mosquito-free zone remained completely healthy. Victory! Because the men had been kept in isolation throughout the experiment, it was clear at last that mosquitoes transmitted yellow fever between humans. Luckily, Moran made a complete recovery.

# THE FUTURE OF YELLOW FEVER

Thanks to the Reed Commission, yellow fever epidemics in Cuba and the U.S. came to an end. Screens and bug repellent help keep mosquitoes at bay, and most people live in cities with water and sanitation systems, so there is less standing water around for mosquitoes to lay eggs in.

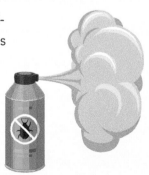

# CLARA MAASS:
# VOLUNTEER OR VICTIM?

Most of the people who volunteered to take part in the Reed Commission's experiments on yellow fever were men—either American soldiers or local Cubans. The lure of $100 in gold was enough to overcome their fear of getting yellow fever. And they were assured of good medical care if they did get sick during the experiments, which was more than they could expect if they contracted the disease on their own.

But at least one woman volunteered for the experiments: Clara Maass. And she wasn't doing it for the money. Clara was an army nurse who had seen firsthand the ravages of yellow fever in the Philippines and Cuba. She wanted to join the fight against the disease.

Clara was bitten by a mosquito that had fed on yellow fever patients. She developed a mild case of yellow fever, from which she recovered. Then, several months later, she agreed to be bitten again, to test whether she had developed an immunity to the disease.

She hadn't. Clara Maass died of yellow fever in the summer of 1901.

Her death caused a massive public outcry in the United States and put an end to yellow fever experiments using human subjects. But as a nurse, Clara Maass understood the risks she was taking. She wanted to be part of the effort to stop yellow fever, even if it meant she lost her own life.

But even today, yellow fever is still a threat in many parts of South America and Africa. Approximately 200,000 people come down with yellow fever each year, and up to 30,000 die from the disease. And that number is growing. The *Aedes aegypti* mosquito, which spreads the disease through its bites, is re-emerging in cities where it has not been seen for years. A small, dark mosquito with white markings on its legs, the *Aedes aegypti* mosquito prefers areas without clean water and sanitation systems.

One scientist in Australia has a plan to wipe out yellow fever and other diseases spread by mosquitoes. Scott O'Neill has bred a strain of mosquitoes loaded with harmless bacteria called *Wolbachia*. The bacteria compete with the viruses, making it harder for the viruses to reproduce inside the mosquito. That makes it much less likely the mosquitoes can spread the viruses to people. O'Neill first released his specially bred mosquitoes in backyards in Queensland, Australia, hoping that they would breed with wild mosquitoes and pass along the *Wolbachia* bacteria to their offspring.

It worked! Dengue fever has almost disappeared from Queensland. O'Neill's World Mosquito Program is now releasing the *Wolbachia*-carrying mosquitoes in countries around the globe.

# VACCINES

In 1936, Dr. Max Theiler, a virologist working at the Rockefeller Foundation in New York, developed the first successful vaccine against yellow fever. Over the next 10 years, the Rockefeller Foundation made more than 28 million doses of the vaccine and distributed them around the world. Theiler, who caught yellow fever himself while working on the vaccine, but luckily survived, won the Nobel Prize in Physiology or Medicine in 1951 for his achievement.

It is often said that vaccines save lives, but it is really *vaccination* that is the lifesaver. A vaccine that stays in the test tube isn't any good at stopping disease. There's a good vaccine for yellow fever, but the fact that people are still getting sick and dying from the disease has more to do with social and economic justice than with science.

To save lives, the vaccine needs to go from the lab to the manufacturer, onto airplanes, across borders, through customs, into warehouses, and then to clinics—and sometimes even right to the homes of the people who need it most. To stop an outbreak, health care workers need to be trained and equipped to deliver the vaccine. Only then can the vaccine do its work of preventing disease.

Vaccination protects the whole community. A disease can't spread from an infected person if everyone around them has been vaccinated and is now immune.

There are now vaccines available for more than 100 infectious diseases.

# MOSQUITOES BEWARE: SHIPS COMING THROUGH

The Panama Canal is one of the world's best shortcuts, giving ships a quick route between the Atlantic and Pacific Oceans. Nearly 14,000 ships use the 80-km (50-mi) canal every year. And it nearly didn't get built—because of mosquitoes.

Hot, swampy, and rainy for much of the year, Panama is a mosquito paradise. But for the canal builders, it was hell. Between 1881 and 1889, more than 22,000 workers died of yellow fever, and by 1906 almost 85 percent of the workers had been hospitalized for yellow fever. To end the epidemic, the U.S. sent Dr. William Gorgas, who had practically eliminated mosquitoes in Cuba after Walter Reed's discovery that they transmitted yellow fever. To get rid of Panama's mosquitoes, Gorgas drained swamps along the canal route, put screens on the windows of workers' homes, and made sure all houses had running water. It worked! The first ship crossed the canal in 1914, just before the start of World War I.

The world's great shortcut also gave a boost to the next great disease outbreak: the Spanish flu pandemic of 1918. Faster travel and increased trade helped the influenza virus spread across the world. It was a pattern that would continue throughout the 20th century and into the 21st: more travel, more trade, more epidemics.

# CHAPTER 4

# COOKING UP TROUBLE

## TYPHOID IN NEW YORK, 1906

"Oh, cook, I just had to come and talk to you about this evening's dinner." Mrs. Warren was rarely seen in the kitchen of the family's grand rented summer house at Oyster Bay, Long Island, and when she did appear, the cook noticed that it always caused a commotion among the staff.

Not surprising, really. Mary had worked for many wealthy families over the years, and in her experience the lady of the house generally came to the kitchen only to complain. She'd been cooking for the Warren family in this fashionable summer resort town for almost three weeks now, so she was probably overdue for a scolding. The clams she'd served tonight—had they smelled a little off? Rich New York City folks could be terribly sensitive, she knew that.

Mary hoped she wasn't going to be fired—it had been hard enough finding this job, and she didn't look forward to the thought of pounding the pavement to look for work again so soon. But to her relief, she realized Mrs. Warren had come to the kitchen to praise her: "The clams were so tender—sublime! And the dessert! So refreshing, just the thing for a warm summer evening. My daughters were in heaven. What do you call that dessert?"

"It's Peach Melba, ma'am. Very fashionable just now. All the best New York restaurants are serving it, they say."

"Peach Melba. How wonderful! You must make it for us again. I am very pleased with you, cook, and I intend to keep you on in the fall. I imagine that suits you?"

"Yes, ma'am. Thank you, ma'am."

"Fine. Good evening, Mary."

# A SHAMEFUL DISEASE

The Warrens' cook, Mary Mallon, went to bed that night glad to have a steady job for the fall. She would happily please her employers with more special desserts. A peach pie, perhaps?

But there would be no more elaborate meals cooked for the Warren family that summer. A few days later, on August 27, 1906, the household awoke to turmoil: Margaret, one of the Warrens' daughters, was seriously ill.

Margaret had gone to bed early complaining of a bad headache. By morning it was worse, and soon she was doubled over with stomach cramps. As the day wore on, Margaret developed a violent cough, and her mother noticed that the girl's skin was hot and dry, almost burning to the touch.

That afternoon, one of the maids collapsed and had to be sent to bed. Then the gardener drooped over his rake, and he too had to be helped into bed. By the evening, the Warrens' second daughter had joined her sister in the sickroom. Finally, Mrs. Warren herself was stricken.

More than half the members of the household were now fighting for their lives. Doctors were called in, first from the nearby town, then specialists from New York City. Private nurses in white uniforms whisked down the corridors, carrying cups of broth on silver trays. There were grave faces, and whispered conferences between the medical men. Finally, the diagnosis was delivered.

Typhoid fever.

Typhoid! It was unthinkable. Wealthy New York bankers' wives and daughters were not supposed to get typhoid, not in 1906. Not in fashionable resort towns like Oyster Bay, Long Island. Typhoid was a disease of the poor. It meant you didn't have proper standards of hygiene in your home. Immigrants, laborers, servants—those were the people who fell ill with typhoid, not the rich and privileged.

Outraged, Charles Warren demanded an explanation from the owner of the summer house, George Thompson. Thompson was worried: If he couldn't find the source of the disease, his luxury summer house might get a bad reputation, and then how would he rent it out next year? If people in New York heard that typhoid was running rampant in Oyster Bay, it could hurt the whole town. And he had four other houses to rent each summer. This mystery needed to be cleared up, quickly and discreetly.

Thompson started asking around for an investigator with a scientific or medical background. A few weeks later, Thompson found just the man for the job: George Soper.

George designed and managed sewer systems for a living, so he knew a lot about how disease could be spread through water contaminated by human waste. He had made a name for himself as an investigator by tracking down the source of a typhoid epidemic in Ithaca, New York, a few years earlier. Now, he packed his bags for Oyster Bay.

The first thing George did was check the house's plumbing. He put colored dye in the Warrens' toilet and flushed it, to see if it would show up in the home's drinking water. The water from the taps remained clear and colorless. Next, he looked for leaks in the home's cesspool, where the waste collected: it was fine. Contaminated milk was a frequent source of typhoid, yet the dairy that supplied the Warren family was spotlessly clean. One by one, George eliminated the usual suspects for a typhoid outbreak. Finding the source wasn't going to be as easy as he had hoped.

George interviewed all the family members, trying to sniff out something unusual that might have happened in the days leading up to the outbreak. Someone recalled that they'd all eaten clams bought from a local woman on the beach. George checked, but none of the clam seller's other customers had gotten sick—it wasn't a case of contaminated shellfish.

Still, it made George wonder if something the family had eaten might have picked up contamination in the kitchen. He went to talk to the kitchen staff, and he heard something that made his ears perk up. The family's cook, hired just three weeks before everyone got sick, had recently quit. He asked more about the cook, an Irish woman whose specialty was a dessert of peaches and ice cream called Peach Melba. Listening to the family sing the cook's praises, George realized that she could have passed microbes to them when she handled the uncooked fruit.

New cook hired. Family gets ill. New cook leaves suddenly without any explanation. It was highly suspicious behavior, in George's opinion. He asked for the cook's name. "It's Mary. Mary Mallon."

# TRACKING THE SUSPECT

George headed straight back to New York City, where he stopped in at an employment agency that supplied the city's wealthiest households with servants. Did they have records for a cook by the name of Mary Mallon? Indeed they did. Working backward through her employment history, George visited each of the families Mary Mallon had cooked for. A disturbing pattern emerged: "In every household in which she had worked in the last 10 years there had been an outbreak of typhoid fever. Mind you, there wasn't a single exception," George wrote in his report about the case.

George's detective work showed that Mary was linked to 22 cases of typhoid and one death—all in homes with no previous history of the disease. But how could Mary have been ill and contagious with typhoid for 10 years? George began to wonder if Mary Mallon was somehow able to pass on the typhoid infection to others without showing any symptoms of the disease herself.

In 1906, a few doctors and epidemiologists were beginning to suspect that, in some cases, healthy people could transmit disease: today they are called "asymptomatic carriers." A German bacteriologist, Dr. Robert Koch, had recently published a scientific paper about a healthy carrier of typhoid. The carrier was a woman who had come down with typhoid years before and made a full recovery. When the doctor examined her, he found to his surprise that her feces, urine, and blood were still full of active typhoid bacteria.

George Soper knew the only way to be sure if Mary was a healthy carrier was to test her urine and feces to see if they contained the *Salmonella typhi* bacteria that caused typhoid. But he had to find her first!

Months went by with no leads. Then, in the spring of 1907, George happened to hear about a family living on fashionable Park Avenue in New York City whose daughter was terribly ill with typhoid. He hurried over and soon learned that the family had recently hired a new cook. Yes, her name was Mary. Why yes, Mary Mallon—did George know her?

George probably ran all the way to the kitchen. He'd found the elusive Mary Mallon at last. But the interview he'd looked forward to for so long didn't go well. In his eagerness to make an important scientific discovery, he overlooked the fact that he was dealing with a human being with emotions, not just a walking collection of typhoid germs.

When a strange man burst into her kitchen and demanded that she give him samples of her blood, feces, and urine, Mary was insulted and horrified. She did what any self-respecting cook would do: she grabbed the nearest weapon—a sharpened carving fork—and chased the madman out.

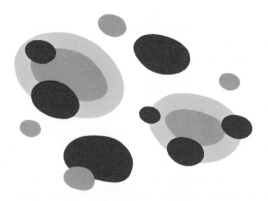

# THE DOCTOR'S PLAGUE

Today, every kid learns about the importance of handwashing. Clean hands are one of the most effective ways of preventing the transmission of communicable diseases. But not too long ago, even doctors didn't bother washing their hands.

When one doctor pointed out that clean hands seemed to help keep patients from dying, his colleagues felt so insulted that they ran him out of the profession. In 1847, Ignaz Semmelweis was working at the maternity clinic of the Vienna General Hospital in Austria. At that time, 10 percent of women who came to the hospital to give birth died from a bacterial infection called puerperal fever. Dr. Semmelweis suspected the doctors were passing the infection from woman to woman, and he asked them to try washing their hands in water and bleach before each delivery. When they did, rates of puerperal fever at the hospital dropped to less than 2 percent. Handwashing worked, but Semmelweis couldn't explain why. When he presented his findings and argued that all doctors should wash their hands, the hospital fired him. He was forced to leave Vienna, and he had difficulty finding work as a doctor ever again.

Twenty years later, Louis Pasteur proved that microscopic organisms cause disease, and suddenly Semmelweis's insistence on handwashing began to seem more reasonable. In the 1880s, when a British surgeon called Joseph Lister started sterilizing surgical instruments, many more people survived operations. Doctors were cleaning up their act.

## TOOL OF THE TRADE: PUTTING DISEASE UNDER THE MICROSCOPE

When George Soper barged into Mary Mallon's kitchen demanding samples of her blood, urine and feces, she must have thought he was out of his mind. In 1907, laboratory tests to identify bacteria in human body fluids were still very new, and the idea that a doctor could diagnose a disease by looking at a tiny blood sample under a microscope sounded ridiculous to most people.

But George Soper's unusual request showed that he was familiar with the most cutting-edge medical developments of his time. Thirty years earlier, the bacteria that causes typhoid, *Salmonella typhi*, had been identified. In 1892, New York City had set up the country's first bacteriology laboratory to investigate threats to public health. George knew that by immersing the samples in a growing medium (often beef broth was used) and waiting 48 to 72 hours, any typhoid bacteria in her urine and feces would be visible under a microscope.

Because Mary had never shown symptoms of typhoid, the new techniques of bacteriology were the only way George could prove that she was the source of the Oyster Bay outbreak. Sure enough, when doctors analyzed Mary's fluid samples, they were teeming with typhoid bacteria.

# ROUND TWO

Unfortunately for Mary, that wasn't the end of it. Very soon, George returned, bringing backup with him.

Dr. Josephine Baker was a medical officer with the New York City Health Department. As one of the city's only female doctors, it was her job to get urine and feces samples from Mary to prove whether or not she was a typhoid carrier. As George Soper had already discovered, it wasn't an easy assignment. When Dr. Baker and two burly New York City policemen showed up, Mary Mallon was suddenly nowhere to be found—and none of the other kitchen staff would tell them where she'd gone.

Josephine and the police hunted through every closet and cupboard in the house, searching for the fugitive. They were ready to give up when the doctor noticed a bit of colored cloth caught in a closed door. It was the edge of Mary Mallon's long skirt, revealing her hiding spot in a tiny cupboard under the stairs.

The doctor and the police had to haul the angry, fighting woman out of the house and into a waiting ambulance. They ignored her when she shouted that she wasn't sick, that she didn't have typhoid, that she'd never been so insulted in her life. Afterward, Josephine remembered how "the policemen lifted her into the ambulance and I literally sat on her all the way to the hospital; it was like being in a cage with an angry lion."

Fecal, blood, and urine samples taken in the hospital confirmed what George Soper had suspected: Mary was a typhoid carrier.

In the early 1900s, 350,000 people in the United States became ill with typhoid every year. In New York City alone, there were more

# DR. JOSEPHINE BAKER:
# PUBLIC HEALTH PIONEER

Mary Mallon and her captor, Dr. Josephine Baker, had quite a bit in common. They were both single women struggling against the odds to make lives for themselves in New York City. Dr. Baker—or Dr. Joe, as she preferred to be called—had the advantage of an education and a medical license, but that doesn't mean she had it easy. In her first year as a doctor, she made just $185—and she had to split that with another doctor who shared her office. To earn more money, she went to work part-time as a medical inspector. That's how she ended up searching for Mary Mallon.

Dr. Joe made many contributions to public health during her long medical career. She was especially interested in the connection between poverty and ill health. In 1907, Dr. Joe was put in charge of the city's new bureau of child hygiene, the first in the country. There, she developed programs that were later picked up in 35 other states: she made sure all children were vaccinated, that free milk was available for children from low-income families, and that people looking after young children got training in the basics of infant care. By 1923, New York City had the lowest child mortality rate of any major city in the U.S., thanks to Dr. Joe.

Epidemiologists continue to explore the question of what makes some people healthier than others, and what policymakers and governments can do to ensure that all people remain as healthy as possible.

than 4,000 cases a year, and the city was trying to clean up its act and reduce the rates of infectious diseases such as typhoid. There were campaigns to clear the streets of garbage, manure, and sewage, and the city was working to establish safe drinking water supplies and sanitation for all its inhabitants.

Typhoid wasn't as deadly as cholera, but it was a very serious disease. A crushing headache and fatigue were the first symptoms, followed by fever, diarrhea, and cramps. It took from two to six weeks of bed rest and medical care to recover from typhoid. A vaccine against *Salmonella typhi* was not developed until 1911, and antibiotics to treat the disease weren't available until 1948. In 1906, all that doctors could do was try to bring down their patients' fevers, watching and waiting for the disease to run its course.

When George Soper started his investigation, no one understood exactly how typhoid spread. We now know that typhoid is caused by eating or drinking something contaminated with the bacteria *Salmonella typhi*. People who have typhoid shed the bacteria in their poop. Other people can be infected by drinking water contaminated with sewage or by eating food that has been handled by an infected person who hasn't washed their hands thoroughly after going to the bathroom. This kind of disease transmission is called the fecal-oral route.

To fight the disease, New York's health inspectors had the right to march into homes where typhoid was suspected. They ordered sick people to stay home, and anyone who didn't follow their orders could be hauled off to a quarantine hospital. Even though Mary wasn't sick, George Soper had proved that she was transmitting typhoid, and the city's health department agreed that it would be dangerous to allow her to continue working as a cook.

So Mary was sent into quarantine, on a tiny island in the middle of New York's East River. Since the 1860s, North Brother Island had been used to quarantine patients with dangerous contagious diseases—smallpox, cholera, yellow fever, tuberculosis. Healthy, strong, able-bodied Mary Mallon was sent to live on the desolate, windswept island, with the sick and dying as her only companions.

# ROUND THREE

Mary fought back—writing letters, demanding her civil rights, and pleading for help to get her released from quarantine. Three years later, the New York Supreme Court agreed to hear her case.

While Mary was on North Brother Island, a surprising thing had happened: 50 other healthy typhoid carriers had been identified, just in the state of New York. Not one of them had been sent to North Brother Island. Health department officials admitted that perhaps they had overreacted. Mary won her case, and her freedom, on the condition that she agree not to work as a cook again. In 1910, after three years as a prisoner of the New York City Health Department, she was allowed to cross the river back to New York City.

The health department didn't see it as their responsibility to train Mary for new work. Instead, they gave her a job as a laundress—one of the hardest, worst-paid jobs for a woman at that time. At first, they checked in with her frequently—then, as the weeks and months passed, less and less regularly. Finally, they lost contact with Mary altogether. What was she doing? Where was she living? It seemed no one cared any longer about the healthy carrier who had caused such a stir only a few years before.

Then, in 1915, a New York City maternity hospital had an outbreak of typhoid. Twenty-five doctors and nurses got sick. Two died. The hospital employment records showed that a new cook had been hired just weeks before the outbreak. The head of the hospital brought in George Soper and showed him a sample of the cook's handwriting.

George knew it right away: "I saw at once that it was indeed Mary Mallon."

Just to be sure, George called Josephine Baker to the hospital. "Sure enough," Josephine wrote, "there was Mary, earning her living in the hospital kitchen, spreading typhoid germs among mothers and babies and doctors and nurses, like a destroying angel."

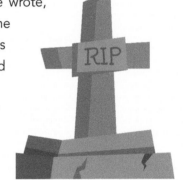

The health department sent Mary back to North Brother Island, where she stayed for the next 23 years. Mary died in quarantine in 1938.

## VILLAIN OR VICTIM?

From the beginning, newspapers had a field day reporting on Mary Mallon's case. When an article in the *Journal of the American Medical Association* in 1908 called her "Typhoid Mary," the tabloids starting using it too. Before long, Typhoid Mary was a household name. Today, we call anyone who spreads disease, intentionally or not, a Typhoid Mary.

Mary Mallon's story still fascinates people. Articles and books and plays and movies have been written, looking for answers to the many questions we still have about her. Did she suspect, before George Soper first approached her, that she might have had something to do with the typhoid that struck all the families she worked for? Why did she risk going back to cooking after she'd finally won her freedom from North Brother Island? Was she a villain? Or was she just an ordinary person whose life was ruined by an uncaring system?

Mary was a woman, a servant, an Irish immigrant to the United States, unmarried, and with little education. All those things meant

# TOOL OF THE TRADE: QUARANTINE

Quarantines have been used for centuries to contain epidemics, by keeping people who have been exposed to a disease separated from the rest of the population, to see if they get sick. The word "quarantine" comes from the Italian for 40 days: *quaranta giorni*. During the plague pandemic of the 1300s, that's how long the city of Venice made ships wait in the harbor before docking, to be sure no one on board had plague.

As the Black Death raced through Europe, other cities began using quarantines. Sometimes entire neighborhoods or towns were sealed off to prevent plague from spreading. But quarantines could backfire. If people in infected cities suspected that a quarantine order was coming, thousands would flee, hoping to get out before they were shut in with the sick and dying. Inevitably, some of the people running away from the quarantine would develop plague, spreading it far and wide.

Quarantine is one of the social distancing measures we still use today to control the spread of disease. In 2020, many countries began requiring anyone returning from an area affected by COVID-19 to self-quarantine for at least two weeks. New Zealand instituted a rule that all travelers must report to a quarantine station and stay there for two weeks, returning to their homes only when they tested negative for the COVID-19 virus.

# THE IRISH POTATO EPIDEMIC

Mary Mallon was one of many Irish people who came to North America in the 1800s and early 1900s. It all started in 1845 when Irish potato farmers discovered their crops were infected with an epidemic of mold: *Phytophthora infestans*.

The potato was the farmers' main source of food, and they couldn't eat the rotten, diseased tubers. A million people starved to death during the potato epidemic. Millions more boarded ships and came to North America to start new lives.

In New York, landlords rented cheap apartments with no running water or sanitation to the new arrivals. Diseases spread quickly in the crowded buildings. Newspaper articles blamed the outbreaks on the new immigrants, and some people said the United States should close its borders. No one pointed their fingers at the landlords or the city government, who were responsible for the living conditions in the buildings. When Mary Mallon, an Irish immigrant, was identified as the spreader of typhoid, it seemed to confirm the idea that new immigrants were sources of disease

When epidemics strike, people still look for someone to blame. Immigrants, LGBTQ+ people, Jewish people, Muslim people, people of Chinese heritage—they've all become targets. The reality is that the pathogens that cause disease don't look for people of a particular race, belief, or sexuality—all they need is a human body to infect.

she had very little power in the society in which she lived. Yet she wasn't afraid to chase officials away, elude doctors, fight the police, swear, argue, and write angry letters until the courts were forced to take notice of her. Doctors and officials were no doubt surprised to see Mary standing up for herself so fiercely, and her behavior may have branded her as a problem case in their eyes.

There's another reason Typhoid Mary's story continues to interest people: it raises questions about how far governments should go when trying to protect the public from epidemics. Was it fair to keep Mary Mallon in isolation for so long? During the SARS epidemic in 2003, the Ebola epidemic in 2014, and again when COVID-19 struck in 2020, people returning from affected areas were ordered into quarantine. Putting people into quarantine, even temporarily, means they may lose their jobs and be unable to provide for their families. Public health officials have to try to balance individuals' rights with the need to protect the public from disease.

## A VACCINE AND A WORLD WAR

Typhoid had killed thousands of troops in the Spanish-American War of 1898. So in 1911, when a British scientist named Almroth Wright developed a vaccine for the disease, army doctors were eager to put it to use. They got their chance during World War I. The vaccine became mandatory for all soldiers in the U.S. army, and the results were impressive: during the Spanish-American War, typhoid had infected 142 out of every 1,000 soldiers, but in WWI that rate fell to less than 1 infection per 1,000 soldiers.

# THE FUTURE OF TYPHOID

If you're lucky enough to live in a city with a working sewer system and a reliable supply of clean drinking water, chances are you've never heard of typhoid fever. In most of North America and Europe, typhoid is a disease of the "bad old days," before engineers, public health doctors, and city planners figured out how to safely dispose of all the human waste generated by cities full of people. But in many parts of the world, typhoid is still a terrifying reality.

The World Health Organization estimates that between 11 and 21 million people get sick with typhoid every year, and up to 161,000 of them—mostly children—die from the disease. At least one in six infected people are asymptomatic and do not realize they are carrying the bacteria that causes typhoid. There are vaccines that can prevent typhoid, but in countries where typhoid is most common, the cost of introducing a vaccination program is too high—as are the costs of ensuring that everyone has access to clean drinking water. Meanwhile, the bacteria that causes typhoid is mutating, producing new strains of typhoid that are resistant to antibiotics: a "superbug." People who develop drug-resistant typhoid stay sick longer and are more likely to be hospitalized, or to die from the disease. In 2016, an outbreak of drug-resistant typhoid emerged in Pakistan, and by 2019 it had infected 11,000 people and caused over 100 deaths.

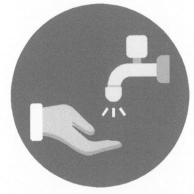

# CHAPTER 5

# WORLD VS. VIRUS

## SPANISH INFLUENZA PANDEMIC, 1918-19

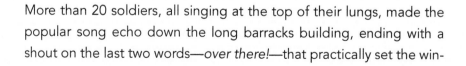

*Over there, over there*
*Send the word, send the word over there*
*That the Yanks are coming*
*The Yanks are coming . . .*
*And we won't come back till it's over*
*Over there!*

More than 20 soldiers, all singing at the top of their lungs, made the popular song echo down the long barracks building, ending with a shout on the last two words—*over there!*—that practically set the windows rattling in their frames. Albert Gitchell's head ached. He pulled his thin blanket over his head and burrowed down in his bunk, trying to block out the noise and get some sleep. In these giant drafty barracks, hastily built only months before to house American soldiers on their way to Europe to fight in World War I, there was no escaping the rowdy songs and laughter that sometimes seemed to go on all night.

There was good reason to stay up singing: it was the only way to stay warm through the frigid Kansas night. Huddled around the glowing stove, clapping hands, stomping feet, sharing cigarettes, the men tried to keep the cold at bay. Normally, Albert would be in the thick of the fun, giving his renditions of all the popular tunes as loudly as he could. But tonight, he longed for quiet. More than anything, he wanted to go to sleep and wake up feeling less achy and feverish than he felt right now.

The winter of 1917–18 was the coldest on record in the state of Kansas. The officers, who would normally order the soldiers to bed, looked the other way and let the men at Camp Funston sing through the freezing nights. It was only the camp medical staff who got angry when they found clumps of men knotted around the stoves for warmth. Then they would lecture the soldiers about the dangers of "spreading contamination." No one paid them any attention. The men needed to keep warm, and if that meant they might spread germs to one another, it was a risk they were prepared to take. After all, what was the worst that could happen—a couple of days in the infirmary?

One of the camp's superior officers had already complained to the army administration about the conditions at Camp Funston, writing that the "barracks and tents were overcrowded and inadequately heated, and it was impossible to supply the men with sufficient warm clothing." The conditions in the camp were perfect for spreading disease. But nothing was done.

Not quite a year earlier, on April 6, 1917, the United States had declared war against Germany, joining the Allied nations—among them England, France, Canada, Australia, and Russia—in the Great War, which we now know as World War I. But the country had only a small army, and they would need many more men to join the war effort. Within a few months, the army had drafted 2.8 million men, and massive camps were hastily erected all over the country to train the new soldiers before they were shipped overseas to the front lines of Europe.

Camp Funston was one of the biggest training camps, but even so, it was crowded. Located in Kansas, it had endless lines of tents and low wooden barracks where 26,000 brand-new soldiers slept and ate and washed together, in spaces designed for far fewer men.

Most soldiers didn't stay long at Camp Funston. They were soon sent off for more training at other camps, or onto ships carrying them to the battlegrounds of Europe. The plan was that by the summer of 1918, the U.S. would be sending 10,000 soldiers to France every day.

And although neither the men singing around the stove nor poor Albert Gitchell knew it, the United States would very soon be sending some invisible cargo to Europe along with its soldiers: a deadly virus.

# THE WARDS FILL UP

Albert woke up early. As an army cook, he was trained to wake up in the pre-dawn hours, long before the reveille sounded, to report for breakfast duty. He dragged himself out of his bunk and dressed in his uniform, even though his body screamed in protest and his head throbbed.

He made his way slowly across the frigid camp to the kitchens. By the time he arrived, the fires had already been lit. He slipped an apron over his head and took his place quietly in the line of cooks, hoping to avoid his sergeant's eye.

An enormous pot of porridge stood in front of him on the range, and he picked up a metal spoon to stir the mess and keep it from burning on the bottom. Nothing made the men complain more loudly than burnt porridge in the morning—that had been one of his first lessons in the army.

*Clang!* The spoon slipped through his fingers and clattered noisily onto the rough wooden floorboards. Wearily, Albert bent down to retrieve it, then turned back to the vat on the stove.

"Private Gitchell! Stop what you're doing right now!"

Albert froze, the spoon in the air above the porridge. It was the sergeant.

"Gitchell, have you or have you not been instructed on the basics of kitchen hygiene?"

"I have, sir," Albert said.

"Then you know better than to use a dirty spoon from the floor. That's the fastest way to get the health officers in here, Gitchell, and we don't want them looking over our shoulders!" As he spoke, the sergeant strode across the kitchen until he was next to Albert. He noticed the young soldier was pale, his eyes glazed. Beads of sweat dotted his forehead. "You feeling okay, Gitchell?"

"Little . . . under the weather this morning, I guess. Didn't sleep too good," Albert replied dully.

The sergeant sighed with irritation. "Hygiene again, Gitchell. Kitchen staff are not to report for duty when sick. Take off that apron and get yourself to the camp hospital."

By the time he had crossed the camp to the hospital, Albert was feeling worse—much worse. The medical officer didn't need to do much more than glance at him before making a diagnosis: "Flu. Report to the contagious ward. You're confined to bed, soldier."

Albert was barely out the door when another man staggered into the hospital. It was Corporal Lee W. Drake of the First Battalion's Transportation Detachment, complaining of headache, fever, sore throat, and aching joints—symptoms identical to Albert's. He was sent to join Albert in the contagious ward. So was Sergeant Adolph Ruby, right behind Drake, also suffering from flu symptoms. Another man followed, then another. The medical officer picked up the phone to alert the camp's doctor about the sudden rash of influenza cases.

When the doctor arrived, he was staggered to see a line of sick men that stretched out the infirmary door and across the hospital grounds. That evening, poor Albert Gitchell was kept awake by noise again—not rowdy singing but coughing and moaning from the more than 100 fellow sufferers crowded into the contagious ward of the hospital with him. By the end of the week, there were 500 soldiers confined to bed with influenza at Camp Funston.

# PRIVATE GITCHELL, PATIENT ZERO

Private Gitchell, army cook, became the first recorded patient in the great influenza pandemic that, over the next year, would kill between 50 and 100 million people around the globe. Albert survived his bout of the flu, but he was one of the lucky ones. At Camp Funston, 48 of his fellow soldiers died from influenza that month, and as the great movement of U.S. troops began, sick men from Funston spread the disease to other camps.

## A VIRUS THAT GETS AROUND

Spanish influenza moved so fast in 1918 that some people thought the disease was the German army's "secret weapon." Or that the disease was released in the clouds of poison gas used on the battlefields.

We know now that influenza is spread from person to person through infected droplets in the air. People with influenza "shed" the virus for three to six days after being infected, often before they have developed any symptoms. And the virus is tough: it can survive on a hard surface like a doorknob for up to two days, waiting for a hand to help it make the leap to a mouth or an eye or a nose.

Influenza is a crowd disease, spreading easily when people are packed together—like soldiers on a troop ship or in the trenches of World War I. Malnutrition, exhaustion, and lack of medical care increase the risk. So many soldiers came down with the flu in 1918, it brought an early end to the war.

In March 1918, 84,000 American soldiers set sail for the port of Brest, in France. In April, 118,000 more boarded troop ships for the journey to the front lines. Influenza spread fast in the crowded ships, and hundreds of men had to be carried off when they landed in France. Thousands more were still walking but extremely infectious. The Allied soldiers already in Europe—British, French, Canadian, and Russian troops—were in weak condition after four years spent in the trenches. Among these men, the influenza virus spread like wildfire.

Tens of thousands of soldiers began filling army infirmaries in the late spring of 1918, too sick to report for duty. And while most were up and around again within a few days, the sheer number of sick men affected military operations. The British navy had to delay launching its fleet for three days that June because there weren't enough healthy sailors available to man the ships.

Soon the virus crossed the no-man's land between the trenches and began spreading among the German troops. For months, Germany had been planning a massive offensive for the spring of 1918, but with tens of thousands of sick soldiers, that operation had to be canceled. Many historians now believe that if influenza hadn't prevented Germany from launching its offensive, Germany might have won the war.

Still, nobody outside the army knew that one of the biggest epidemics in human history was underway. Almost every country had a wartime censorship law that put restrictions on what newspapers and radio stations could report. Printing or broadcasting any news that could hurt the war effort or damage public morale—making people worry that their own country wasn't going to win the war—was forbidden. So letting people know that hundreds of thousands of soldiers were sick was definitely off-limits.

That meant members of the public didn't take precautions that might have kept them from catching the disease, like staying away from crowds. Instead, people were encouraged to attend rallies and parades in support of the troops. The disease spread fast among the civilian population in Europe. Even the king of Spain came down with a case of influenza. Spain, unlike almost every other country in Europe, wasn't involved in the war. It was officially neutral, so its newspapers were free to print all the news. That spring, the big news in Spain was the influenza epidemic. Other countries, unable to report on their own epidemics, reprinted the articles about the outbreak in Spain, and so the disease that spread across the world came to be known as "Spanish influenza."

## IT WASN'T "JUST THE FLU"

Doctors had never seen anything quite like Spanish influenza. Some of the first major outbreaks happened at military camps near Boston in the early fall of 1918. In a letter to a friend, one camp doctor described the horrors he was witnessing: "Two hours after admission they have the Mahogany spots over the cheekbones and a few hours later you can begin to see the Cyanosis [a condition in which the skin turns blue from lack of oxygen] extending from the ears and spreading all over the face. It is only a matter of hours then until death comes and it is a struggle for air until they suffocate. It is horrible. We have been averaging about 100 deaths a day, and still keeping it up…It takes special trains to carry away the dead. For several days there were no coffins and the bodies piled up something fierce, we used to go down to the morgue & and look at the boys laid out in long rows. It beats any sight they ever had in France after a battle."

# CALL IN THE SCIENTISTS

Soon, influenza was out of control, causing chaos and death around the world. And there didn't seem to be anything doctors could do to stop the spread of the disease or to help its victims. U.S. Surgeon General Victor Vaughan commented bitterly that the doctors of the day "knew no more about the flu than 14th century Florentines had known about the Black Death."

It was a big setback. Until Spanish flu came along, medical science had been making steady progress in the fight against disease. Cholera, typhoid, yellow fever, malaria: many of the terrifying diseases of the past could now be effectively treated. Then suddenly this new, deadly strain of influenza appeared and began decimating populations worldwide. And it was happening with such lightning speed that there was almost no time for the scientific community to come up with solutions: no time to develop vaccines, no time to organize a worldwide public health response.

In the U.S., one team of scientists was working hard to analyze the spread of the disease. On April 18, 1918, the head of the Public Health Service sent a letter to Dr. Wade Hampton Frost, asking him to take charge of the newly formed Office of Field Investigations of Influenza. It was a grand title for a small operation with very little funding. Wade Frost had previously investigated typhoid outbreaks along the Ohio River and polio epidemics in New York. He was one of the most respected American scientists in the new field of epidemiology.

# THE SECOND WAVE HITS

For Wade and his small staff—he had just one other full-time doctor working with him, and a few clerks and assistants—the task at first seemed overwhelming. Then, before they'd even been able to put together a research strategy, it looked as if their problems might be over. In early summer, the flu suddenly vanished—or seemed to. The hospitals and the army's infirmary tents were no longer overrun with flu sufferers, and life returned to normal for soldiers and civilians. But it didn't last long: the virus was mutating, or changing its form. It was soon to reappear as an even deadlier disease.

# A NEW SCIENCE FOR A NEW CENTURY

"You're an epi-what?"

Epidemiologists are used to getting blank looks when they tell people what their job is. In 1918, Dr. Wade Hampton Frost's job description probably left most people scratching their heads. Epidemiology was brand new at the time, and almost unknown.

In 1850, a group of British doctors and statisticians had formed the London Epidemiological Society to study epidemic diseases in the context of public health. But it took another 30 years before the British government hired the first epidemiologists to oversee public health and investigate disease outbreaks. In North America, things moved even more slowly: it wasn't until 1902 that the U.S. Public Health Service was founded, and it was another 10 years before Harvard University opened the first school of public health in 1913.

When Wade Hampton Frost was asked to conduct epidemiological studies on the 1918 influenza epidemic, it was a big step forward for epidemiology. It was also a step into the unknown. No one had ever done a study of the size and scale needed to understand the path of Spanish influenza through the United States. Wade and his small team needed to develop methods for gathering and analyzing vast amounts of data, well before computers existed. Their success helped usher in an era of using epidemiological approaches to fight and prevent some of humanity's most feared diseases.

In a single week that fall, influenza epidemics exploded in three cities around the world: in the African city of Freetown, Sierra Leone; in Brest, France; and in Boston, U.S. These three outbreaks launched the second wave of the pandemic. Over six terrible weeks in the fall and early winter of 1918, tens of millions of people would get sick, and millions would die of influenza.

All three cities were major transport hubs for the military. American troops passing through Brest picked up the virus and distributed it around Europe. Soldiers returning home to North America passed through Boston to board the trains that carried them—and the virus— to every corner of the continent. Ships on their way between Europe and battlefields in Africa and the Far East stopped in Freetown to take on coal to fuel their engines—and throughout the fall of 1918, they also brought along the influenza virus.

## WILL THIS WORK?

There was no cure for Spanish flu, so people turned to folk remedies to protect themselves. Garlic, mothballs, sugar lumps topped with kerosene, pills of powdered cinnamon, and eucalyptus oil were all used to try and keep the flu away. Some people thought a potato in your pocket could keep you healthy, while others ate raw onions to repel the germs.

Con men sold "sacred pebbles" supposedly blessed at a shrine in Japan to ward off Spanish influenza. You could also try sprinkling sulfur on your shoes or inhaling the smoke from smoldering wet hay. Many people thought that smoking tobacco would ward off infection. One store in Holland made smoking compulsory for its employees.

Of course, none of these methods stopped the Spanish flu. In fact, by making people feel that it was safe to go out in public, folk remedies like these may have led to *more* people catching influenza.

The pandemic caused a crisis in many countries because of the wartime shortage of doctors and nurses. In the U.S., a third of the doctors and nurses in the country were involved in the war effort, and those who remained to care for the civilian population were overworked and undersupplied. Even when a flu victim could find a doctor or an available hospital bed, there wasn't much that could be done to treat the disease. Doctors relied on rest, liquids, and hope to pull patients through. All too often, patients didn't make it.

No one had ever seen influenza like this before. Patients could develop any of an array of extreme symptoms: terrible pain; very high fevers; chills; earaches; headaches lasting for days; bleeding from the nose, mouth, ears, and eyes; vomiting of blood; and lungs so filled with fluid that patients almost literally drowned. Often, before death, patients turned blue from a lack of oxygen to the blood—what one doctor described as "a dusky, leaden hue."

The disease could overtake you so quickly, there were reports of people dropping dead in the streets, and of people who went to bed at night healthy and were found in the morning stone-dead. There were stories of entire families falling sick, and of children left orphaned and alone in homes filled with the dead bodies of their families. Some cities ran out of coffins, so the dead had to be buried in mass graves. Horse-drawn wagons went up and down the streets, the drivers calling for people to bring out their dead. Scenes like these had not been seen since the days of the Black Death, when plague decimated the population of Europe.

As this new strain of flu swept the world, wartime media blackouts had to be abandoned. Across the United States, Canada, and Britain, governments and media warned people to protect themselves. Movie theaters, dance halls, libraries, restaurants, and churches—

anywhere that people might congregate—were closed. Posters and signs advised people to cover their faces when coughing or sneezing, and many people took to wearing gauze surgical masks over their faces.

But nothing, it seemed, could stop or slow down the spread of the disease. In Dublin, Ireland, public health workers poured huge amounts of disinfectant into the street gutters in an attempt to protect the city. New Zealand began to hunt down all the rats in its towns and cities, in case they were the culprits in spreading influenza. These and other misguided attempts had absolutely no effect on the pandemic.

Tragically, late that fall, the second wave of the pandemic got a huge boost from an unexpected event: the end of the war. When peace was declared at 11:00 a.m. on November 11, 1918, massive celebrations broke out all over the world. City centers were jammed with celebrating crowds, impromptu parades took place, people laughed and shouted and sang, they hugged and kissed and shook hands—and they spread influenza.

## WHAT'S IN A NAME?

To Hungarians, the disease was known as the "Black Whip." Germans called it *Blitzkatarrh* (lightning cold) or "Flanders Fever." In Poland, it was known as the "Bolshevik Disease," and in Spain it was "Naples Soldier." People in Ceylon named it "Bombay Fever." The Swiss called it *La Coquette* (the courtesan), Italians knew it as "Sandfly Fever." To the Japanese, it was "Wrestler's Fever," while in France it was *La Grippe* (the flu). But if you were British, Canadian, or American, the disease that had everyone terrified during the fall of 1918 was the "Spanish Flu."

The names might have been different around the world, but almost all of them had one thing in common: they directed the blame for this dreadful disease at someone else.

# AN INFLUENTIAL REPORT

As the second phase of the pandemic started, Dr. Frost and his small research team struggled with a tidal wave of information. Data poured in from locations all over the world where influenza outbreaks were being reported. And there were major inconsistencies in the reports. In some cases, influenza was reported as a cause of death, while in others death was attributed to pneumonia. Were those deaths part of the pandemic too?

Part of the confusion came from the fact that U.S. doctors treating influenza patients in 1918 were not required to report the cases to the local board of health. Influenza, up until then, had not been considered a disease that the Public Health Service needed to track—unlike diseases such as smallpox, typhoid, or cholera, which they were very concerned about and kept close tabs on. Who had needed to track the number of cases of flu, which was usually a mild three-day illness?

For Wade Frost and his team, this lack of information presented a major difficulty. How could they determine how widespread the disease was, or how lethal it was, without knowing how many cases there were? The only answer was "shoe-leather epidemiology," going house to house, knocking on doors, asking how many in each home had suffered the flu and how many had died. It was the same technique that John Snow had used in London during the 1854 cholera outbreak.

Wade had conducted shoe-leather surveys himself in New York, while investigating a polio outbreak there in 1916. But how could one small office survey an entire country, much less the entire world, to track the course of a pandemic?

In the end, Wade knew he could only hope to survey a tiny sample. He and his team chose 10 cities, then trained hundreds of canvassers, who they sent out to interview the inhabitants. Over the spring of

1919, the surveyors talked to 112,958 people, asking them in detail about their experiences during the Spanish flu pandemic. Had they gotten sick? Did they know anyone, a friend or neighbor or family member, who had come down with influenza? How long were they sick for? What were their symptoms?

## IT'S A MUTANT!

Influenza is a master of disguise and very changeable. We can develop vaccines to protect us, based on the versions of the virus we already know and predict might be heading our way again. But every time a new strain of the flu emerges, our immune systems fail to recognize it, and new flu vaccines have to be formulated. Scientists call these changes to the virus "mutations." And thanks to these ongoing mutations, we get sick with flu year after year.

Influenza viruses can mutate in two ways: through either "antigenic drift" or "antigenic shift." (An antigen is any substance, like a toxin or a virus, that causes an immune response in the body.) Antigenic drift is a process of gradual change, in which the virus changes bit by bit. Antigenic shift is fast and causes big changes. Scientists speculate that antigenic shift caused the Spanish influenza virus to turn lethal in the fall of 1918.

In August 1919, Wade published his report on the pandemic. Called "The Epidemiology of Influenza," it contained two important discoveries that are still studied by epidemiologists. First of all, the report noted that before anyone was aware of the influenza epidemic, there had been a rise in the number of reported deaths from pneumonia. Since pneumonia is a lung infection that can result from influenza, an increase in pneumonia is one of the early warning signs of a flu epidemic that public health agencies still look for today. The report also demonstrated that influenza was a particularly lethal killer of the very old and the very young—which is why flu vaccinations are now given first to people over age 60 and under 5.

The 1918 influenza pandemic also killed an unexpectedly high number of healthy young people, and its path of destruction came to be known as the "lethal W" because charts of the death rates showed an alarming bump in the middle. Why did Spanish influenza kill so many people who were in the prime of life? It's a riddle that has continued to fascinate medical researchers. Scientists now estimate that a similar strain of flu had not appeared for at least 70 years before the 1918 epidemic, so almost no one had any immunity to Spanish influenza. That meant that many more young adults came down with Spanish influenza than would be expected in a normal flu outbreak.

But this was no normal flu, either: it was deadly. Some researchers believe that the Spanish influenza virus triggered an overreaction in its victims' immune systems. The strong immune systems of healthy young people were turned into killing machines by the virus, causing such extreme symptoms that the sufferers eventually died.

## HOW MANY DIED?

We'll never know exactly how many people caught Spanish flu and how many died of the disease. Epidemiologists estimate that the death toll may range anywhere from 50 to 100 million. That's a big range.

Between 16 and 18 million people may have died in India alone. (Spanish flu also came hard on the heels of a plague epidemic that killed 12 million people in India between 1898 and 1918.) While there are no statistics available for countries in Africa, estimates place the number of deaths in the tens of millions. There are also no reliable statistics for the death tolls in Southeast Asia, China, or South America. In Canada, 50,000 people died from Spanish flu, while in the U.S. there were 550,000 deaths. In Britain 228,000 people died, in Germany 400,000, and in France 300,000.

# TOOL OF THE TRADE:
# FINDING PATIENT ZERO

Wade Hampton Frost made one of his biggest contributions to epidemiology long after the Spanish flu pandemic. In the 1930s, Wade was investigating abnormally high rates of tuberculosis in the U.S. state of Tennessee. Tuberculosis is an infectious lung disease that kills millions of people worldwide every year.

As he pored over the records of cases, Wade realized that when an outbreak could be traced back to a single individual, the full pattern of the outbreak could be reconstructed. Finding this person would allow epidemiologists to determine how the disease was spreading, how contagious it was, and what made people vulnerable to the disease. He called that person at the center of the outbreak the "index case." Epidemiologists still use the term, as well as the techniques that Wade developed to identify the index case.

Today, we sometimes also call the first person to get a disease, "patient zero," a term that became popular after it was used in a book about the spread of AIDS in the US.

# COLD CLUES

For many years, there was no way to study the virus that caused Spanish influenza. The mystery of what had made the disease so deadly was buried along with its many victims.

Then, in the 1950s, a researcher at the University of Iowa got the idea of looking for the virus in the Alaskan permafrost. Johan Hultin learned that an isolated village in Alaska, Brevig Mission, had been almost entirely wiped out by the Spanish flu: 72 of 80 residents had died in 1918 and were buried in a mass grave. Johan realized that the bodies might be preserved in the permafrost. If he could get a tissue sample from one of the victims, it might be possible to isolate the virus that had killed them. Johan got the permission of the village elders to open up the grave, and he traveled to Alaska to start digging.

He recovered frozen tissue samples, but to study them he had to get back to his lab in Iowa. He started the long trip home, stashing his precious samples in airport refrigerators and hotel freezers in between flights to try to keep them from thawing out. But by the time he returned, the samples were ruined and he was not able to extract the virus. With no money to return to Alaska, Johan was forced to give up his dream of solving the mystery.

Johan was already retired when in 2005 he heard about a research team that had developed a new method to isolate genetic material from tissue samples. He leapt at the chance to return to Brevig Mission to finish what he'd started 50 years before. This time, the researchers successfully reconstructed the virus. They were able to determine that the Spanish flu was caused by an avian (bird) virus, and they developed a vaccine, making the world safe from another Spanish flu pandemic.

# LESSONS FROM THE SPANISH FLU

More than 100 years after the end of the worst pandemic in history, scientists are still studying the records of Spanish flu to understand how it spread so far, so fast—and what worked to slow it down. There was no effective treatment, so controlling the spread of the pandemic depended on what epidemiologists now call "non-pharmaceutical interventions" or NPIs. These are things like staying home, washing your hands, staying a safe distance from others when out, wearing a mask, and avoiding large gatherings.

In early 2020, as COVID-19 infections spread around the world, public health officials told people to follow the same rules that had worked in 1918. With no vaccine or cure for COVID-19, NPIs were the best way to stay safe. Schools and businesses closed. People stayed home, going out only to buy food. But not everyone agreed on how long it needed to continue. Did the experience of cities during Spanish flu offer the answers?

Epidemiologists who have studied the data from 1918 agree that timing was important: cities that acted fast to shut down places where people gathered, such as churches, theaters, and schools, had lower infection rates and fewer deaths. But when those cities relaxed the rules, influenza came back. Scientists comparing the epidemic curves of different cities during the 1918 pandemic noticed that in places where people continued to practice social distancing, there was no second wave of infections. The conclusion: the key to surviving the Spanish flu was to go home and *stay* home.

# SOCIAL DISTANCING:
# AN OLD IDEA IS NEW AGAIN

In 2005, a new book about the Spanish flu pandemic was published. Called *The Great Influenza*, it told the story of how the virus spread around the world in the final years of World War I. Heading off for vacation that summer, the president of the United States, George W. Bush, tossed *The Great Influenza* into his suitcase, thinking it would be an interesting read about a long-ago time.

Instead, his summer reading got him thinking about the future. President Bush came back from vacation and told his staff that they needed to start planning. How would the United States handle a future pandemic like the Spanish flu?

The answer, it turned out, was not new. The scientists who were called on to come up with a plan used modern science to prove that social distancing methods first used in the Middle Ages—like quarantine and self-isolation—were the most effective ways to prevent the spread of illness.

These days, many people expect that whenever they get sick, their doctor can prescribe a drug to cure or treat the illness. It seemed like, with the advice to just stay home, medical science was taking a step backward. But in fact, scientists were applying lessons learned from the Spanish flu epidemic and using state-of-the-art computer modeling to prove that social distancing works.

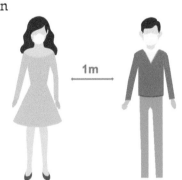

1m

# THE START OF SOMETHING NEW

The huge numbers of people who were infected and killed by Spanish flu convinced health officials and governments around the world that they had to make changes to the way medical care was delivered. At the time, most doctors worked for themselves, or for charities or religious organizations. They weren't required to report cases of disease to the authorities, so there wasn't an easy way to tell that the pandemic was coming.

Over the next few decades, country after country started offering their citizens free health care, or socialized medicine. Norway was the first, followed by countries like Japan, New Zealand, Britain, France, Germany, and Canada.

The spread of the flu across the globe proved that international cooperation was needed to control disease, so in 1919 the first international bureau for fighting epidemics was formed. It would eventually become the World Health Organization, which in 2020 took the lead in the fight against COVID-19.

# A GOOD HOST

Spanish influenza was a strain of avian (or bird) flu that spread to the human population. Wild aquatic birds are the "host species" for avian flu: the virus occurs naturally among them. Occasionally, an infected wild bird may spread the disease to a domesticated bird, like a chicken, duck, or goose. From there it can make the leap to people.

Many flu epidemics have started where people live in crowded conditions and in close contact with poultry. In 1997, a type of bird flu spread from nearby poultry farms to Hong Kong, China. Public health officials, worried that another lethal influenza pandemic might start, killed all the poultry in Hong Kong and the surrounding area—as many as 1.5 million birds!

In 2003, the bird flu came back. There were small outbreaks of highly pathogenic avian influenza, commonly called H5N1, in China, Korea, Vietnam, Japan, and Thailand, but only people who were in direct contact with poultry became sick. The World Health Organization reported that by 2020 there had been only 861 confirmed cases of H5N1 in people, and 455 deaths. But will the virus mutate and spread from human to human, starting yet another pandemic? That's a question that worries scientists.

# CHAPTER 6

# MYSTERY IN THE JUNGLE

## EBOLA IN ZAIRE, 1976

The room was stuffy and windowless. Paint was peeling off the walls, leaving damp, scabby patches of discolored plaster. But the floor was clean, and so was the narrow iron cot in the corner. A man lay on the cot, sweating. His eyes were glazed. The only sound was a faint wheeze as he panted for breath. Mabalo Lokela was very sick.

It was September 1976, and Mabalo was in Zaire, a country of steamy, sprawling jungle and congested cities in Central Africa. Zaire, now known as the Democratic Republic of Congo, was not a good place to be sick. The country was still recovering from almost a century of brutal colonial rule by Belgium. Under colonialism, all the profits from Zaire's rich natural resources—rubber, ivory, and diamonds—went to the wealthy Belgian landowners. Meanwhile, the Zairean people had labored in the mines and the rubber plantations for low wages, forced to live in poverty without schools, hospitals, good sanitation, or clean water. Even after the country won its independence from Belgium in 1960, there was political instability, and the country fell under the rule of a powerful dictator. Zaire struggled to recover, and there weren't enough doctors, nurses, clinics, or drugs to treat everyone needing medical help.

Mabalo's hometown, in Zaire's remote northern Équateur province, was a particularly unlucky place to fall ill. Yambuku was surrounded by jungle, hours away by rutted dirt road from the nearest town. The village had no doctors—just a clinic run by an order of Catholic nuns.

Mabalo, the village schoolteacher, was just back from a hunting trip with family and friends from the surrounding villages. Now he had a raging fever, a splitting headache, and a body racked with cramps. Malaria, he was pretty sure. Mabalo had been ill with malaria before. Mosquitoes bred in the low wet fields cleared for coffee plantations, and since no villagers could afford screens on their windows, everyone was vulnerable to the "shaking fever."

He lay in one of the Yambuku mission's examining rooms. He hoped that the nuns might have some drugs left over from their last shipment of supplies from Europe. He'd get a shot, go home, and hope that the fever receded enough so that in a week or two he could work again.

The nun who bustled in to treat Mabalo agreed that, yes, it seemed he'd got malaria again. Sister Beata wasn't a nurse—none of the missionaries had any formal medical training—but she'd seen many cases of malaria. She filled a glass syringe with the antimalarial drug chloroquine (pronounced klor-uh-kween) and gave Mabalo the injection he'd been waiting for. Soon, he was making his slow way home, leaning heavily on his wife M'buzu's shoulders.

At first, it seemed as though Sister Beata's injection was working, as it had many times before. But after a day or two, Mabalo's fever returned with a vengeance. Soon, he was too weak to get up, and his body was ravaged by terrible bouts of diarrhea and uncontrollable vomiting. His wife and two oldest daughters struggled to care for him. Neighbors took in the younger children as the crisis in the family's hut deepened. In desperation, M'buzu begged the nuns to visit her husband, hoping they might be able to cure him.

When the sisters entered the family's small hut, Mabalo was lying on a low bed. He was covered in sweat and gasping for breath. Patches of dark blood were spreading from his ears and pooling beneath his nose and eyes. As they stared, terrified by the change that had come over him, Mabalo convulsed and vomited a stream of blackish blood.

M'buzu turned to the frightened nun beside her. "Sister, can you help? Do you have any medicine that will cure him?"

Slowly, Sister Beata shook her head. "This is new," she said quietly. "This is definitely new."

The virus that had infected Mabalo was causing his internal organs to disintegrate into a soupy mess that seeped from his orifices and through his skin. With every retch, Mabalo released millions of infectious microbes into his surroundings. Every blood-and vomit-soaked rag his daughters washed was a time bomb of lethal microorganisms. Sister Beata was right: this disease was new, and it was very dangerous.

# HELP US!

For seven long days and nights, the nuns and M'buzu fought to keep Mabalo alive. But at last he was claimed by the nightmarish illness.

Surrounded by her children, and helped by her family members and neighbors, M'buzu began preparing her husband's body for the funeral. Together, the group carefully washed the body, sponging away the thick-crusted blood. They would sit with the body all day and all night before carrying Mabalo to his grave just outside the family's hut.

As the wails of mourners reverberated through the hot, still air, the nuns, gathered in prayer in the mission's tiny church, felt a sense of relief. Mabalo's terrifying illness was over. Life could return to normal in the village and the mission.

But a few days later, everyone began getting sick.

Mabalo's wife, his eldest daughter, his mother, his sister, and his mother-in-law were the first to come to the mission clinic suffering from fever, headache, vomiting, and diarrhea. More followed. Within days, 21 people who had attended Mabalo's funeral were showing symptoms of the same violent illness. Others in the village, and throughout the surrounding area, were falling ill as well.

The nuns, with their limited knowledge of medical procedures and scanty supplies, struggled to comfort the dying. Then they too began dying. Sister Beata was among the first.

In the mission office, Sister Marcella, the Mother Superior, hunched over the shortwave radio sending out message after message to the outside world, pleading for help. The fever was spreading fast, and it killed almost every person it touched, young or old, healthy or frail.

For the nuns, for the grieving families, for the villagers numb with fear, there were so many questions. What was causing this terrible disease? Why had it chosen to strike their village? How was it being it spread, and how could the living protect themselves from this killer?

# A MICROSCOPIC QUESTION MARK

As the first of October dawned in Yambuku, the epidemic was in its third week. Already, well over 100 people were dead. Alerted by Sister Marcella's calls for help, doctors from Zaire's capital city, Kinshasa, arrived to collect blood samples that they would analyze to try to identify the mystery illness.

There were no longer enough living staff at the mission to care for the sick and dying. Sister Marcella sent the remaining patients home and ordered the mission's gates to be chained shut. The nuns gathered together in the chapel to pray and wait for death.

With no clinic to care for the sick, fever patients were taken to neighboring villages to be cared for by family members—spreading the infection throughout the region. Village elders warned people to stay home. Schools and shops closed, social gatherings were discouraged, and trees were felled to block the roads, preventing travel between villages. Almost overnight, the epidemic zone became a network of ghost towns.

Meanwhile, the blood and tissue samples the Kinshasa doctors had collected were being studied around the globe. Scientists were peering into microscopes and realizing with a jolt of fear and excitement they were looking at a virus that had never been seen before.

In Belgium, 27-year-old Dr. Peter Piot, a researcher in the microbiology lab at the Prince Leopold Institute of Tropical Medicine, was one of the first to look down the barrel of a microscope at the virus. He soon realized the mysterious microbes were lethal: laboratory mice injected with tiny amounts died within days. Doctors in Zaire had suspected the disease might be related to yellow fever, but all the antibody tests were coming up negative. With its curved, whiplike tail, Peter thought the virus looked like a question mark—a question mark taunting him and his colleagues.

When the director of the institute told Peter that the World Health Organization (WHO) was sending an international team of scientists to Zaire, Peter didn't ask to go—he demanded to be sent as Belgium's representative. This deadly virus was a question, and he was determined to find answers.

# ON THE HUNT

Days later, sitting on a flight to Kinshasa, Peter started to wonder what he'd gotten himself into. Seated next to him was a Belgian diplomat who was furious that an inexperienced young doctor was part of the team fighting the mysterious killer disease: "Intolerable! We're facing a terrible epidemic, and all they could find is you? How old are you? Twenty-seven? You're totally green, you're barely even a doctor. You've never seen Africa in your life!"

The taxi ride from the airport through Kinshasa didn't help to calm his growing nervousness. Everywhere he looked there were throngs of people, and the sticky heat and humidity had him panting. He'd hardly been out of Belgium before, and never anywhere as unfamiliar as this city. Had he been foolish to sign up for this mission?

The hastily assembled group of scientists knew they needed more information. They decided to send a scouting team to Yambuku to investigate the epidemic and try to find out how it was spreading. Who was willing to volunteer?

Before the question was even finished, Peter had his hand up.

# MEET THE MICROBE

"Watch out, I've got a nasty virus. You don't want to catch it."

We've all heard that before. But what exactly are viruses?

A virus is a type of microbe, or single-celled organism. Microbes are the oldest and most numerous life-form on earth, and they are essential to human life.

There are several types of microbes, including bacteria, fungi, viruses, and the lesser known archaea and protista. Without microbes, we couldn't digest our food, breathe, or break down wastes. But some microbes cause potentially lethal diseases—like Ebola.

Viruses are the tiniest, and in many ways the strangest, of all the types of microbes. Scientists can't even agree whether viruses are alive. Until a virus comes into contact with a host cell, it is nothing more than a lifeless bundle of DNA. But once it makes contact with cells in your body, the virus springs to life, hijacking the cells and using them to reproduce itself and spread. Illnesses from the common cold to AIDS and Ebola are all caused by viruses. And many of the symptoms of viral illnesses—such as coughing, vomiting, diarrhea—help to spread the virus to new hosts.

# COLLECTING CLUES

*"Yaaaa!"*

Peter choked from the searing pain in his throat. Around him, a circle of men laughed uproariously. As soon as his eyes stopped watering, Peter joined in the laughter.

It was his first taste of arak, a powerful homemade alcohol popular in Zaire. As Peter was discovering, sharing a drink of the fiery liquor with the community leaders was a good way of gathering information about the epidemic.

He had arrived early that morning in Yalikonde, the nearest village to Yambuku. As he stepped from the jeep, he was struck by the brooding silence. No children played in the central square, no adults lingered to gossip outside the huts, no shops were open. At first, only a few people ventured out to talk to the foreign doctor.

But later, as the cup of arak was passed around, the elders began to tell him about the outbreak in their village. They brought Peter into the huts of the sick so he could see the suffering the disease inflicted on its victims. As frightened as he was, Peter felt useful in a way he never had while working in the lab in Belgium. He took blood samples and interviewed family members, noting the names of the dead, when they had died, and their relationships with other fever victims.

By visiting every village within driving distance of Yambuku, the scouting team determined that over 200 people had died of the fever, and there were still infected victims.

# FROM SOCCER TO FUNERALS

Each night when the WHO team members returned to their headquarters at the Yambuku mission, they shared the data they had collected and the notes they had taken. Soon the scientists had enough information to plot graphs of the disease, showing the number of cases by location, age, and gender, and the dates of known deaths. To everyone's relief, the graphs indicated that the worst of the epidemic was probably already over.

The scouting team was doing its job: collecting enough information so that a full-scale investigation could be set up in the region. But Peter was frustrated. He wanted to find answers to the questions that were tormenting him. How was the disease being transmitted? Why had it spread so quickly from Mabalo Lokela to the rest of the village? And where had the virus come from?

One evening, Peter drove to the village of Yamotili-Moke. The village elders welcomed him, and soon a lively debate about the strengths and weaknesses of Belgian and African soccer players started. Peter stayed and talked through the evening, and he returned again the following night. Unlike the systematic data-gathering he did during the day, during these conversations Peter took no notes. He just listened, piecing together information about local customs and culture. He wasn't sure how this would help to fight the epidemic, but he knew that if he wanted to help these people, he needed to understand them better.

Peter's instinct soon proved right. One evening, the conversation turned to the preparations for the latest fever victim's funeral, and as they spoke, Peter learned why a pattern of new infections followed each funeral. It was customary for family members to honor a deceased person by washing the body and sitting with it overnight before burial. These practices meant that there were many opportunities to come into contact with infected blood and body fluids. Peter immediately advised the elders to put a stop to their customary funeral rituals for fever victims.

# TOOL OF THE TRADE:
# QUALITATIVE RESEARCH

When Peter Piot arrived in Zaire, he had no formal training as an epidemiologist. Very few people at that time did. Aside from a few internationally recognized organizations, such as the U.S. Centers for Disease Control and Prevention in Atlanta, Georgia, there were hardly any research laboratories in 1976 that specialized in epidemiology. That meant scientists learned epidemiology on the job.

The investigative team sent to Zaire took blood samples, drew detailed maps of epidemic-stricken areas, asked the same questions of people over and over again, and noted down everything. But Peter Piot realized that in addition to the "how many" approach of quantitative research (for example, finding out how many people had come into contact with each patient, and how many of those people got sick), the researchers needed to add the element of "why." They needed to uncover why some people were getting infected while others weren't. And that meant spending time with villagers to learn the details of their everyday lives.

That kind of approach is called qualitative research. As Peter wrote years later, "It's like detective work. You take blood samples also, but the essence is…talking, talking, talking…and understanding."

As he reviewed the data they'd collected, Peter noticed something else that worried him. A high number of young women were contracting the disease. Usually in an epidemic, more deaths were to be expected among the very old or the very young—those without reserves of strength to fight the disease. But in this case, it looked as though those most vulnerable were women between 18 and 25. The number of deaths of young women was more than double that of young men. What could be the explanation?

Peter recalled what he'd learned about the activities at the Yambuku mission clinic before the epidemic had forced it to close. Despite a tiny staff and only the most basic equipment and supplies, the mission had served the medical needs of thousands of people throughout the region, including offering prenatal care for pregnant women. Peter was willing to bet that many of those expectant mothers were between the ages of 18 and 25. Could there be a connection between the mission and this terrible epidemic?

Peter knew he needed to get a look at the clinic for himself.

# CRACKING THE CASE

As Peter toured the empty rooms with Sister Marcella, he told her about the high number of deaths among young women. Had anything unusual happened at the mission's prenatal clinic, he asked, around the time that Mabalo Lokela fell ill?

Sister Marcella smiled as she remembered those happier days, when the mission's courtyards had been filled with the bustle of patients and families. She told Peter proudly about the excellent prenatal care that young mothers received at the clinic, and in particular the popular weekly vitamin shots. All pregnant women visiting the mission clinic were given an injection of vitamin B12.

# NAME THAT VIRUS

Laboratory scientists today can choose from a few different methods of identifying a virus. One of the oldest methods, first developed in the early 1900s, is to grow a "culture" of the virus. A scientist places a small sample of the infected blood or tissue in a cup, along with cells in which the virus can grow—the "culture." As the microbes grow in the culture, changes in the cells will be visible under a microscope. By observing these changes, the scientist can identify the virus or bacteria that is causing the disease.

In 1890, German scientist Robert Koch suggested four guidelines for scientists to follow, to help them determine if an infectious organism (such as a virus) is the cause of a specific disease. These rules, still followed by scientists today, are now called "Koch's Postulates." A scientist must be able to answer "yes" to each of the following questions before concluding that a virus causes a particular disease:

1. Is the organism found in people with the disease and absent in people without the disease?

2. Can the organism be grown from blood or tissue samples taken from a person sick with the disease?

3. When the organism is given to a healthy person, do they develop the disease?

4. Can the organism be grown again, from blood or tissue samples from this second person?

With a growing sense of dread, Peter asked to see where the drugs and medical equipment were stored. In the clinic's small dispensary, he opened drawers and cupboards one after another. Finally, he turned to Sister Marcella.

"There are only five syringes here for the entire clinic. How did you manage to give so many injections with such a small stock?"

The sister replied matter-of-factly that each morning the syringes were sterilized. After that, they were used over and over again for all the patients treated that day, with a quick rinse between uses. On their meager budget, she explained, the clinic couldn't afford to buy more syringes or needles.

Peter realized with horror that the nun who had given Mabalo Lokela his shot of chloroquine had unwittingly spread the infection to every pregnant woman in the village through the unsterilized needle. Here was the link he'd been searching for. The epidemic had been spread by the very clinic to which people had turned for help.

Peter carefully bagged two of the syringes to take back to Kinshasa for testing. "I'd bet anything these are both infected," he thought sadly to himself.

The scouting team's findings were correct: the epidemic had spread through unsterilized needles and through contact with infected patients in the mission clinic and at funerals.

The last infected patient died on November 5, and there were no further cases reported. The international scientific delegation continued to work in Zaire for several months, collecting more information about the mysterious disease that they began to call Ebola, naming it for a nearby river.

# WHERE DOES EBOLA COME FROM?

Peter Piot's team never learned how Mabalo Lokela contracted Ebola, but we now know it is transmitted to humans through contact with infected animals. The Ebola virus has been identified in gorillas and chimpanzees in Africa, and scientists think that, in at least some outbreaks, the index case—patient zero—was either a local hunter or a customer who bought infected meat from hunters.

Gorillas aren't the reservoir species for the virus (where the virus lives in between the human outbreaks), because Ebola kills gorillas almost as fast as it kills humans. The evidence currently points to African fruit bats as the reservoir species. Fruit bats may infect humans directly or transmit the virus to them indirectly, through other animals.

The key to preventing future outbreaks of Ebola is reducing the risk of animal-to-human transmission. That may sound simple, but it isn't. Here are some of the reasons why Ebola outbreaks are continuing in Africa:

- Disappearing forests: Logging and farming are putting more people into formerly wild areas, and into contact with animals.

- War: Refugees fleeing from wars often have to hunt for food.

- Climate change: Habitats are changing, and some animals are moving closer to human settlements.

- Poverty: There aren't enough hospitals or doctors in some areas of Africa.

# THE ROAD AHEAD

Researchers identified the Ebola virus as a filovirus—one of only two ever discovered. The filoviruses are a small family of viruses causing extremely lethal diseases in humans and other primates. Both the filoviruses, Ebola and Marburg, cause severe hemorrhagic (pronounced hem-or-rhag-ik) fever—illnesses in which the victims bleed profusely. Ebola kills 88 percent of its victims, making it one of the most lethal diseases on the planet. In the Yambuku outbreak, 318 people were infected and 280 died.

Between 1977 and 2020, there were 29 Ebola outbreaks in Africa and elsewhere, including 3 in the U.S. Four workers at U.S. research facilities in Virginia and Texas who were accidentally bitten by monkeys developed Ebola antibodies in their blood—proteins produced by their immune systems in response to the Ebola virus. But the workers never developed symptoms, although the monkeys became sick with Ebola and most died. This particular strain of Ebola, which is not dangerous to humans, was named Ebola-Reston, after the city in Virginia where it was first identified.

At the time Ebola emerged in 1976, medical science seemed to be winning the war against disease, with powerful weapons like vaccines and antibiotics in their medical arsenal. Ebola reminded everyone of the vast number and diversity of disease-causing viruses and bacteria, and of how much scientists and doctors still had to learn about fighting disease.

# HOT LABS

Microbiology laboratories around the world use a numbering system to identify their level of "biosafety"—the degree of risk that is involved in working at the facility. There are four levels. In Level 1 labs, scientists work only with organisms that do not cause disease. In Level 2 labs, mild disease-causing microbes can be handled. Level 3 labs work with serious diseases for which treatments or vaccines exist. Only in Level 4 labs are the most lethal, highly infectious, and untreatable diseases allowed.

To get clearance to study life-threatening microbes, Level 4 labs must create "hot zones": isolation chambers located either in a separate building or in a highly controlled area within the main lab. Before entering a hot zone, researchers dress in special coveralls, over which they pull a bright blue, heavy-duty pressurized hazmat (hazardous materials) suit equipped with a breathing apparatus called a Chemturion. Before entering and after leaving the hot zone, the researcher must also pass through a series of decontamination showers, a vacuum room, and an ultraviolet light room, in order to eliminate all potential traces of disease.

# ANIMAL DISEASE DETECTIVES ON THE CASE

On March 23, 2014, the World Health Organization confirmed that an epidemic of Ebola had broken out in Guinea. Seven days later, epidemiologist Fabian Leendertz was on a plane, heading to Guinea to try to discover the cause of the epidemic. Fabian is a wildlife epidemiologist, a specialist in investigating outbreaks of disease in animal populations.

Other outbreaks of Ebola in humans have been linked to epidemics in animals, such as gorillas, chimpanzees, and small antelopes called duikers. The disease spreads to humans when hunters kill and butcher infected animals. But in the village of Meliandou, the first people to die of Ebola were two-year-old Emile and his mother, grandmother, and sister. That was a clue that the virus had originated in a smaller species, one that makes its home close to human populations. Like bats.

Fabian already knew that some bats could carry the disease without getting sick, including fruit bats that live in the forests of Guinea. If he could prove that the outbreak had spread from bats, people in the region could be warned to stay away from the animals. That could help to prevent further infections.

After four weeks of surveying the forests around the village of Meliandou, capturing bats and testing them, Fabian still hadn't found any infected animals. Then he heard some intriguing news: villagers told him about a hollow tree, near where Emile and his family had lived, where bats used to roost. The tree had burned down shortly before the investigators arrived, but Fabian suspects that Emile could have been bitten while playing in the hollow tree, or become infected through bat droppings.

# THE BAT CONNECTION

Take an evening stroll in a large city in Africa, Australia, or South Asia, and you may spot something unexpected fluttering through the night sky, dodging between the skyscrapers and high-rise apartments: bats. Most of the furry flying mammals are newcomers to cities, and they haven't come by choice. In some cases, their forest homes were cut down as people built new settlements or cleared land for farms. Others have ended up in cities when the changing climate forced bat colonies to move in search of food, abandoning the forests in favor of nesting near human settlements

All around the world, bats and people are living closer together, in bigger numbers, than ever before. That's bad news for the bats, and it also spells trouble for humans. Because of their unique body structures and genetics, bats are ideal carriers for viruses. The viruses don't make the bats sick, but if the bats spread the virus to other animals, the result can be devastating. Ebola is one example of a virus spread by bats that has caused epidemics in gorillas, chimpanzees— and humans. The coronaviruses that cause SARS and COVID-19 may also have spread to humans from bats.

Veterinary epidemiologists are realizing that to prevent new diseases from emerging to infect humans, we need to take an eco-system approach to health—one that considers the links between weather patterns, wildlife health, and humans. When humans disrupt an ecosystem, they increase the chances that a pathogen will jump from wildlife to us. Since the middle of the 20th century, the human population has expanded and the climate has gradually warmed up, causing unusual rainfall patterns that affect the availability of food for

# THE WOMAN WHO SAVED A COUNTRY

In December 2013, the largest Ebola outbreak ever spread from Guinea into Sierra Leone, Liberia, and Nigeria. That's where it found Patrick Sawyer, an American visiting his sister.

Patrick's sister was one of the first to die of Ebola. Afterward, Patrick was desperate to get home to Minnesota. He never made it.

Patrick collapsed in the airport and was rushed to the hospital. Although he was shaking with fever, he demanded to be released so that he could fly home. Dr. Stella Adadevoh was the doctor in charge that day, and she was alarmed by Patrick's symptoms. "Close off this ward," she ordered. "Get masks, get gloves. All we have." She called the public health authorities to tell them she had an Ebola patient in her hospital.

When Patrick learned that Dr. Adadevoh wouldn't release him, he ripped the IV line from his arm, spraying blood over the floor, and tried to escape. Two days later, Patrick was dead and the doctor was fighting for her life, along with 19 other hospital staff infected with Ebola. In the end, Stella Adadevoh died, one of eight people killed by Ebola after coming into contact with Patrick Sawyer. If not for her quick thinking, the virus could have started spreading among the 21 million people in Lagos, Africa's biggest city. She may also have saved the United States, where Patrick was headed. She put herself at risk, telling Patrick Sawyer and the other doctors and nurses that it was "for the greater public good."

In 2014, the World Health Organization declared that Nigeria was Ebola free. But the epidemic raged for another two years in surrounding countries, infecting 28,000 people and killing 11,000. Ebola outbreaks continue to occur in Africa.

animals. When animals have to change their habits in order to find food, it often brings them into closer contact with other species, and with humans. Environmental scientists warn that this could lead to more virus exchanges between animal species, increasing the likelihood that another virus will jump to humans.

# EBOLA'S PATH TO PATIENT ZERO

Scientists have put together a picture of the environmental conditions that led to the start of the 2014 West African Ebola outbreak, using data from weather satellites high above Guinea.

A long drought had recently ended with weeks of heavy rains. At last, the orchards and plantations that surrounded the towns and villages of Guinea were full of fruit. The scent of the ripe fruit lured hungry animals out of the forests, and apes and bats crowded under the trees to feast. Fruit bats are messy eaters, and they would have scattered half-eaten fruit on the ground. An ape, picking up a discarded piece of fruit, could have ingested a pathogen from the bat's saliva or droppings along with his juicy lunch. And once the virus started circulating in apes, the chances increased that the virus would find its way to humans through hunting.

## ZOMBIES!

Seen a good movie or TV series lately? How about *The Walking Dead*, a popular show about a group of pandemic survivors on the run from zombies? Or *World War Z*, *I Am Legend*, or *Train to Busan*? Every year there are new movies about epidemics that threaten to wipe out human life and turn us all into bloodthirsty hordes of zombies.

Zombies (or at least the idea of them) have been around in folklore for hundreds of years. Their popularity on our screens these days tells some researchers that people are looking for safe ways to explore their fears about infectious diseases, especially as we become aware of how quickly a disease can spread. The Centers for Disease Control and Prevention even decided to get in on the act, starting a Zombie Preparedness Campaign to build awareness about how to prepare for emergencies—like a zombie apocalypse.

# CHAPTER 7

# THE NEW PLAGUE

## AIDS PANDEMIC, 1980

Michael sighed and shifted in his seat, searching for a comfortable position. He crossed his legs, uncrossed them, turned, twisted, slumped so his head rested on the seat back—then straightened up again irritably. It was just no good. He'd been sitting on this hard plastic bench, in this stuffy room, for hours. He felt terrible, and he was pretty sure that at this rate he was going to be spending his whole night here, in the emergency waiting room of the University of California, Los Angeles (UCLA) Medical Center.

He looked around. Since he'd first walked in, the faces in the waiting room had hardly changed. There was the old man with the rattling cough, over in the corner was the anxious couple with the crying baby, next to them was the young man holding the bloody bandage around his hand. Not one of them looked like the glamorous jet-setters he'd imagined himself among when he made the big move to Los Angeles a few years ago.

Feeling lost and alone, Michael wondered if he'd done the right thing by moving to L.A. Did he really belong here, in this big, faceless city? Back in his hometown, whenever he got sick, he could drop by his family doctor's office and count on getting a thorough checkup right away.

Michael reminded himself that he'd come to L.A. for good reasons. Number one, he'd always dreamed of making it big as a model, and that wasn't going to happen in his small hometown. And number two, he was gay. He wanted to live where he could be himself, not hiding or masking his true feelings.

In 1980, being LGBTQ+ was tough—there weren't that many places where you could count on a community of people to support you. In L.A. he'd met other young people like himself, who'd come to the big city from small towns across 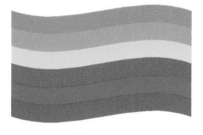 the U.S. They'd all taken big risks. Many had left behind families and friends who didn't understand or accept them. He'd formed close friendships in L.A. and built a new life for himself.

"Michael? Is there a Michael here?"

Michael shook himself out of his stupor, realizing with a jolt that the bored and weary nurse with the clipboard was actually calling his name. "Yes! Yes, I'm coming."

He struggled up out of the plastic seat, dismayed at how weak and dizzy he felt. The nurse flicked open a curtain and ushered him into the first cubicle, motioning for him to sit up on the edge of the high hospital bed. When he'd seated himself, she rattled back the curtain and vanished, the words "Doctor'll be here soon" coming faintly through the thin green drape.

Michael prepared himself for another epic wait. But it wasn't long before the curtain swept open again, revealing a white-coated medical resident—a doctor in training. The resident listened closely as Michael described his symptoms, scribbling notes and nodding. The sore throat, for weeks now; the difficulty swallowing; the weakness and fatigue; the fevers; the weight he couldn't stop losing. Michael tried to joke about it: "I'm so skinny now, I can't even get modeling jobs. Too thin to model—that's got to be a first!"

The resident paused in his note-taking to study his patient. Michael looked like a model, all right, with high cheekbones, bright blue eyes, and short blond hair. But his arms and legs were like sticks, deep shadows were carved under his eyes, and he struggled for breath. This young man was very sick. The resident made up his mind.

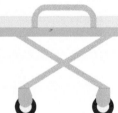

"If you don't mind waiting some more, I'd like to call in a colleague on your case. An expert. We may need to run some tests."

# A PUZZLING SITUATION

Somewhere on Dr. Michael Gottlieb's desk, the phone was ringing. But where?

The doctor scrabbled frantically through the piles of paper—research reports, medical files, lecture notes—until he found the phone. He pulled it up through the layers, yelling, "Hello, hello! Gottlieb here!" before it even got close to his face.

Michael Gottlieb had been working as an assistant professor of immunology at the University of California, Los Angeles, Medical

Center for four months. He hadn't managed to do any filing, but he had convinced his residents and students to keep their eyes open for patients who showed symptoms of uncommon diseases. So when his phone rang late that January evening in 1981, he guessed that it might be a report of an interesting new case.

What he heard from the resident on the other end of the phone soon had him running down to the emergency room.

Dr. Gottlieb discovered that Michael's sore throat was caused by a severe case of thrush. Thrush is an infection of the mouth, throat, and tongue, caused when the fungus *Candida albicans* accumulates on their surfaces. Dr. Gottlieb wouldn't have been surprised to see thrush in a young baby with an immature immune system, or in a cancer patient whose immune system had been weakened by chemotherapy drugs. But why would Michael get thrush? He was an apparently healthy young man, with no history of immune system problems. And what about his weight loss? Was that connected to this mysterious infection somehow?

Dr. Gottlieb was intrigued—and worried. When Michael told him he'd been feeling exhausted and feverish for weeks, Gottlieb decided to admit Michael to the hospital while he searched for the cause of his illnesses.

As Dr. Gottlieb would remember afterward, "It was just such a striking, dramatic illness, and he was so critically ill. It was a distinctly unusual thing for someone previously healthy to walk into a hospital so significantly ill. It just didn't fit any recognized disease or syndrome that we were aware of."

For a first step, Dr. Gottlieb decided to give Michael a blood test. When the results of that test landed on his desk, he decided to go talk to his patient.

Michael was in bed, looking even thinner and paler than he had just a few nights earlier in the emergency room. The doctor sat down beside the bed and tried to smile. "Michael, we've found something kind of unusual. You've got a very low white blood cell count. Do you know what that means?"

Michael looked at the intense young doctor and joked: "Well, I guess that must mean that I'm a 100 percent red-blooded American male."

Gottlieb laughed appreciatively. "Oh, sure. Definitely. But here's the thing, Michael. If we think of your body as an army, then the white blood cells are the advance troops, sent out to detect and take down enemy invaders. They defend you against infections. Without white blood cells, your immune system can't do its job. That's why you've got this bad case of thrush—your body isn't defending itself the way we'd expect. And until we can figure out why your immune system is having so much trouble, you're at risk of getting more infections."

Michael nodded slowly, staring down at the sheets as Gottlieb spoke.

"Your case is a bit of a puzzle so far," the doctor continued. "But I like puzzles, and I'm going to solve this one."

# BAD NEWS

Dr. Gottlieb prescribed antibiotics to clear up the thrush, and Michael was discharged from the hospital and sent home to recuperate. But a few weeks later, he was back in the emergency room, even sicker than before. As Gottlieb had predicted, a new infection had slipped past Michael's weakened immune system—the doctor suspected he now had pneumonia.

Michael lay motionless, too weak to do much more than listen, as the doctor delivered the bad news.

"Michael, you've got a kind of pneumonia called *Pneumocystis carinii*. It's pretty rare. And you've also got another infection, a cyto-megalovirus, or CMV, infection. That's what's making you so tired and weak. Both of these are what we call opportunistic infections—viruses that aren't normally a threat to healthy people. They've attacked you because your immune system is so weak right now.

"And," the young doctor confessed, "we still can't figure out why."

# A PATTERN EMERGES

Only a few weeks later, Michael died. Gottlieb was no closer to solving the puzzle, but he was determined to keep looking for answers.

Meanwhile, across town, another doctor had a patient with a list of symptoms that didn't make sense. Dr. Joel Weisman was gay, and so were many of the patients who came to see him at his North Hollywood office. One patient, a young gay man, had recently come to Joel complaining that he was tired all the time, had swollen lymph glands, kept getting fevers, and was losing weight—more than 14 kg (30 lb) in just a couple of months. The man was getting sicker by the day, but Joel couldn't figure out why. He decided to refer the case to an immunologist, and he called up Michael Gottlieb.

As Dr. Gottlieb listened to his colleague describe the patient, he had only one thought: "Michael!" Sure enough, blood tests revealed that this patient had a CMV infection and hardly any white blood cells. Soon, just like Michael, the young man developed *Pneumocystis carinii*. Not long after, he died.

Could two deaths from such similar causes be simply a strange coincidence? Michael Gottlieb didn't think so, and his hunch was right: three weeks later, he learned that a third patient with the same symptoms had been admitted to hospital in L.A. This case was a replica of the first two: a CMV infection, a low white blood cell count, a lung infection. A pattern was emerging. All three men were young and healthy but had severely damaged immune systems. All three of the men were also homosexual. What was making these young men so sick? Whatever it was, it was lethal.

Michael Gottlieb started calling around to other hospitals and doctors in California, asking if they had seen any cases of CMV infection or *Pneumocystis* recently. A hospital in Santa Barbara had, and they sent him their records on the case. When Dr. Gottlieb read that the patient in Santa Barbara was gay, he knew that puzzle pieces were starting to fall into place.

He decided to get in touch with an old friend from medical school, Dr. Wayne Shandera. Wayne was L.A.'s chief disease watcher, an epidemic control officer with the Epidemic Intelligence Service.

Michael Gottlieb told Wayne what had been happening in the past few weeks. Wayne hadn't heard of anything that could be making young men in L.A. sick, and he felt the deaths might be coincidental. But when a report landed on his desk the next day about a man from nearby Santa Monica who had been diagnosed with *Pneumocystis* pneumonia, he decided to check it out.

He discovered that the patient was 29 years old, with no history of immune system problems, and he was gay. When tests showed that the patient also had a CMV infection, Wayne called his friend Michael Gottlieb and told him that he had just found a fifth case.

# TOOL OF THE TRADE:
# EPIDEMIC INTELLIGENCE SERVICE

When Dr. Wayne Shandera wrote his article describing the first five cases of what would later be called AIDS, he was taking a two-year training program through the Epidemic Intelligence Service (EIS), still run today by the U.S. Centers for Disease Control. The EIS is the medical equivalent of the Central Intelligence Agency, or CIA—but the enemies EIS agents hunt down are biological.

Every year, top medical and scientific graduates in the U.S. are accepted into the EIS program. They're sent to cities all over the country to investigate suspicious outbreaks. For two years, they are on 24-hour alert, ready at a moment's notice to travel to the latest epidemic hotspot. The logo of the EIS features a shoe with a hole in it, over a map of the world. It's a reference to the "shoe-leather epidemiology" pioneered by John Snow, and that's the way these epidemiologists still work: going from door to door in the middle of an epidemic to get the information they need to stop the outbreak.

Today, there are programs like the Epidemic Intelligence Service in 36 countries, with more in development. EIS trainees and officers like Dr. Shandera work to prevent all kinds of threats to public health.

As Dr. Gottlieb later recalled, "A shiver went down my spine. With just a little bit of information, [Wayne] was able to go right out and find a case." The two doctors suspected they were seeing the beginnings of an epidemic.

To be sure, they needed to let other doctors know about the cases in L.A. That June, they published an article about Michael and the other patients in *The Morbidity and Mortality Weekly Report*, a medical journal from the U.S. Centers for Disease Control and Prevention (CDC).

Soon, the phones at the CDC headquarters in Atlanta started ringing with calls from doctors in New York, New Jersey, and San Francisco. Within a month, the CDC knew of 15 young men around the country who had developed *Pneumocystis*. They'd also heard about 26 cases of young men with Kaposi's sarcoma, a rare form of skin cancer. All the patients were gay.

Over the summer and fall of 1981, doctors at the CDC kept hearing about men struggling with unexplained weight loss, rare forms of tuberculosis, unusual cancers. In New York, San Francisco, and other cities with large LGBTQ+ communities, rumors spread about the deadly new disease some people were calling "gay cancer."

Epidemiologists at the CDC had no idea what was causing the epidemic. Was it sexually transmitted? Did it come from food, or from a drug? Was it contagious, like a cold or the flu? No one knew, and people kept dying.

## SOLVING THE PUZZLE

All the patients who had been seen so far were men. But not all LGBTQ+ men were getting sick. So, what was the determining factor? To find out, researchers at the CDC decided to perform case-control studies, which would compare patients to "controls"—individuals who shared many characteristics with the patients but were healthy.

# PIECES OF THE PUZZLE

In 1981, two CDC epidemiologists started knocking on doors, just as John Snow had done more than a century before, talking to the people who were suffering from the new and mysterious collection of symptoms. Mary Guinan and Harold Jaffe criss-crossed the country, visiting hospital rooms, asking everything they could think of that might establish links between the cases and reveal what was causing the illness. Between the two of them, they talked to more than three-quarters of the people in the U.S. who had come down with the disease so far.

The two epidemiologists asked people to describe what they ate, where they had traveled recently, what kind of work they did. Did they have pets? Was there a history of cancer in their families? Had they served in Vietnam, and possibly been exposed to chemical weapons? One after another, they ruled out the possibilities.

They began to suspect that this new disease was transmitted in the same way as hepatitis B (a liver infection caused by a virus), which was through sexual intercourse or sharing needles. But there was a third way that people could develop hepatitis, which they hadn't seen yet in any of the patients they'd interviewed: through blood transfusions. If the new disease was transmitted through bodily fluids, would it show up in donated blood that was stored for patients who needed transfusions? Before long, they had the answer. In 1982, a hemophiliac who had received a transfusion from a blood bank developed symptoms of the disease.

In Los Angeles, New York, and San Francisco, 180 men agreed to take part. Researchers probed into the men's daily lives, health, and backgrounds, looking for clues to what was making some of them sick while others remained healthy.

But even before the studies were completed, it became clear that it was not only LGBTQ+ men getting sick with the new disease. The CDC began hearing reports of other patients with depressed immune systems and opportunistic infections. Hemophiliacs were one new group of patients. Hemophilia (pronounced heem-o-fill-ee-ah) is a rare condition in which a person's blood doesn't clot. People with hemophilia may bleed uncontrollably from even small cuts and scratches, so they often require blood transfusions and blood products that help their blood clot normally. Was the disease transmitted through infected blood? Other new patients included people who used illegal drugs they injected into their veins, like heroin. Doctors knew these drug users often shared needles, which could explain how the disease was spreading among this group.

The evidence was pointing toward a virus transmitted between people through bodily fluids. The researchers at the CDC realized that it was a disease with the potential to go global: anyone could become infected. And doctors had no way to treat it.

# THE EPIDEMIC WITH NO NAME

By the end of 1981, 270 cases of this new disease had been identified in the United States, and 121 of the patients had died. Early in 1982, the disease began to be reported in a number of European countries. And in Africa, doctors in Uganda made a connection between the reports from the U.S. and patients they were seeing who were suffering from an illness known locally as "slim." Slim was a fatal disease that caused severe weight loss, infections, and unusual cancers. It didn't

# CALLING FOR CHANGE

LGBTQ+ people in all parts of the world have long faced legal and social discrimination. In the late 1970s and early 1980s, there was little protection for the rights of the LGBTQ+ community. There were laws in the U.S. against homosexuality, forcing many people to remain "in the closet," afraid to share their lives with their families and communities.

In 1979, 100,000 LGBTQ+ people marched in Washington, D.C., in the first ever National March on Washington for Lesbian and Gay Rights. Governments began passing laws to outlaw discrimination on the basis of sexual orientation.

Attitudes changed more slowly than laws, however, and when AIDS appeared, fear of the deadly disease increased the stigma against LGBTQ+ people. Because of the danger of AIDS, more and more LGBTQ+ people in North America and other parts of the world started to stand up for their rights and to call on governments for action in the fight against the disease. Without the activism of many committed LGBTQ+ people, public education campaigns about AIDS would not have happened, research would not have been funded, and many more people would have died.

take long to figure out that slim and the "gay cancer" from the U.S. were one and the same. The new disease, doctors began to realize, was already a massive global epidemic.

Unless you were a doctor or an LGBTQ+ man living in the U.S., though, you probably didn't even know that a terrifying new disease was spreading. None of the major TV networks had reported on the story. It wasn't until June 17, 1982, that *NBC Nightly News* featured a story on a "new deadly disease" affecting gay men. And it was almost another year—May 1983—before the *New York Times* newspaper ran a front-page article on what scientists were calling Gay-Related Immune Deficiency. By that time, the epidemic had been going on for nearly two years, with over 1,400 diagnosed cases in the U.S. More than 500 people had died.

Every day, more LGBTQ+ activists demanded that this story— about the terrible disease killing their friends and loved ones—had to be told. Their slogan was "Silence = Death." In cities across North America, England, Australia, and Europe, LGBTQ+ groups started offering counseling, food, and support to people suffering from the disease.

Slowly, their activism worked. Instead of "Gay-Related Immune Deficiency," the disease became known as AIDS—Acquired Immuno-deficiency Syndrome. In 1987, researchers in France and the U.S. were recognized for discovering the virus that causes AIDS. They named the virus HIV, for human immunodeficiency virus. With the virus iden-tified, doctors could begin testing patients' blood, allowing for earlier diagnosis than had been possible before. If a patient was carrying the virus, they would be identified as "HIV positive."

But back in 1982, scientists were still making progress slowly, learning more about what caused AIDS, how it spread, and who was most at risk. And to

# WHO WAS PATIENT ZERO?

In 1987, an American journalist named Randy Shilts published a book entitled *And the Band Played On: Politics, People, and the AIDS Epidemic.* It was an instant bestseller, and Randy Shilts became a media sensation.

The book investigated the reasons it had taken so long in the U.S. for the AIDS epidemic to get attention and funding from government and public health agencies. It also told the story of an early AIDS patient called Gaetan Dugas. Gaetan, a French-Canadian flight attendant, participated in the case-control study run by the Centers for Disease Control and Prevention. It turned out that Gaetan was the only connection linking many of the patients. He'd infected the others through unprotected sex.

To maintain his privacy, the CDC study identified Gaetan in their records as "Patient O," the "outside of California" case. Of course, the letter O looks a lot like a zero, and some people assumed that it meant this case was the source of the outbreak. Shilts found Gaetan's name and called him "the man who spread AIDS from one side of the continent to the other." *Time* magazine ran a story headlined "The Appalling Saga of Patient Zero," and suddenly the AIDS epidemic had a new villain—someone to blame for the terrible disease that had everyone so frightened.

We know now that Gaetan Dugas, who died in 1984 of AIDS-related kidney failure, didn't single-handedly cause the AIDS epidemic. But in the 1980s, finding someone to blame was one way for people to make sense of this terrifying, unstoppable epidemic. Just like Typhoid Mary in the New York outbreaks of typhoid, people saw this patient zero as a villain who made others sick through irresponsible behavior.

slow down the spread of the epidemic, they needed help—from governments and from the media. That help was slow to come.

AIDS had first appeared in groups of people—LGBTQ+ men and drug users—who were considered "bad" or immoral by many others at the time. In the early 1980s, lots of LGBTQ+ people tried to keep their lives a secret, fearing that otherwise they would face violence and risk losing their jobs, their homes, their families. As AIDS emerged, that situation seemed to get even worse.

Prejudice against LGBTQ+ people kept governments from funding research into AIDS. Prejudice kept the media from reporting on the epidemic for fear of offending the public. The Centers for Disease Control and Prevention decided not to fund sex education programs that included instructions on how to avoid AIDS through safe sex. The U.S. government refused to fund AIDS awareness materials if they "promoted" LGBTQ+ "lifestyles." To change these attitudes, LGBTQ+ people realized that they had to organize, advocate, and demand the funding that was needed to save lives. They formed organizations to buy AIDS medications and distribute them to patients in need. They shared information, wrote newsletters, held demonstrations, and fought for the money to fund research to save their friends who were dying from the disease.

At last, governments and media began to respond to the AIDS crisis. In some parts of the world, public health information on AIDS became more widespread, and campaigns to promote safe sex appeared, along with much greater media attention. But the death toll for the AIDS epidemic continued to mount. People who had received blood transfusions were at risk, and many hemophiliacs, including children, developed AIDS. Babies with AIDS were born to mothers who had the virus. With each passing year, the tragedy of AIDS deepened. It was not until 1985, when more than 6,800 people in the U.S. had already died of the disease, that the president of the United

# DISCOVERING THE VIRUS

The virus that causes AIDS was discovered in 1983 by Françoise Barré-Sinoussi, Luc Montagnier, and Jean-Claude Chermann at the Pasteur Institute in Paris, France. The three French scientists took tissue samples from the lymph nodes of people with AIDS. They grew the virus in the laboratory from these samples and identified it using an electron microscope.

A team of American researchers led by Dr. Robert Gallo identified the virus at around the same time, and for years, the two countries disputed which group of scientists had been first to make the important discovery. There was a lot at stake: the American government had registered a patent for an AIDS test based on detecting the presence of HIV, and if it was proven that the French team had discovered the virus first, the money from that patent would go to France.

In 1987, the two countries negotiated a settlement: they would split the proceeds from the patent 50-50. Twenty-one years later, in 2008, the French scientists were awarded the Nobel Prize in Physiology or Medicine for their discovery of HIV.

States first said the word "AIDS" in public. The next year, there were 12,000 deaths. By 1988, the yearly total had reached 20,000. By the end of the 1980s, AIDS had become a deadly pandemic.

# THE FUTURE OF AIDS

By the end of 1985, every region in the world had reported at least one case of AIDS, with 20,303 cases in total. In the first 50 years of the AIDS pandemic, nearly 75 million people were infected with the HIV virus, and approximately 35 million died of AIDS. In 2019, 1.7 million people acquired HIV.

Of the 38 million people living with HIV in 2020, more than 25 million were in Africa. In 2018, an estimated 470,000 people died of AIDS-related deaths in the region. In some parts of Africa, about 1 in every 20 adults has HIV. Millions of children have lost their parents to AIDS.

Some of these children are raised by their grandparents. Sometimes the older children in the family are left alone to care for the younger ones. Finding food, clothing, and shelter can be a terrible struggle—and because these children have no opportunity to go to school, their chances of getting out of poverty are very slim.

Today, we know that AIDS can be transmitted only through the exchange of bodily fluids, and there are ways to prevent the transmission of AIDS and stay healthy. Practicing safe sex by using condoms during sexual intercourse is one important preventive measure. Not sharing needles is another.

Thanks to education and prevention campaigns in many countries, far fewer people today are becoming infected with HIV. And doctors have developed a number of drugs, collectively called highly active antiretroviral therapy (HAART), that help to bolster immune systems in HIV patients so that they don't develop opportunistic infections. There are more antiretroviral treatment programs in African countries than ever before, thanks to a huge focus on making this treatment afford- able and widely available over the past decade. More than 62 percent of the people living with HIV in Africa currently receive antiretroviral drugs.

## JUST THE FACTS, PLEASE

The terms AIDS and HIV are often used together, but there are some import- ant differences in what they mean. HIV, or human immunodeficiency virus, is the virus that causes AIDS. When a person becomes infected with HIV, the virus attacks their body's white blood cells, reproducing inside each cell and destroying it, then moving on to the next one, until the person's immune sys- tem is in tatters. AIDS—acquired immunodeficiency syndrome—is the final stage of HIV infection, when the immune system has become so "deficient" that it can no longer protect the body from infections. At this stage, people begin to suffer from opportunistic infections, such as Kaposi's sarcoma or *Pneumocystis carinii*. Eventually, they die from these illnesses.

Today, people infected with HIV can take antiretroviral medication to slow down the rate at which the virus reproduces in their bodies. With antiretroviral therapy, people with HIV/AIDS can avoid opportunistic infec- tions, stay healthy, and live much longer.

However, some people may still not seek treatment because they are ashamed of being HIV positive. People with HIV may face discrimination and stigma. In one survey in Ethiopia, 50 percent of people said they would not buy food from someone if they knew the person was HIV positive. Another 42 percent said they didn't think children with HIV should go to school.

Scientists are warning that the COVID-19 pandemic could have a terrible impact on AIDS patients around the world. Disruptions to services and supplies because of the shutdowns in many countries may mean that millions of people lose access to antiretroviral drugs that suppress the virus and keep them healthy. There could be as many as 500,000 additional deaths from AIDS in 2021 as a result.

# THE STIGMA OF AIDS

In the 1980s, when AIDS was first reported in the media as the "new plague," many people panicked. There were lots of rumors and false information—for example, that you could get AIDS from kissing someone with the disease, or by sharing food with them, or drinking from the same glass. Even some medical personnel were afraid to touch people with AIDS. Some people were afraid that anyone who was LGBTQ+ might potentially have the disease. LGBTQ+ men themselves grew terrified as more and more of their friends fell ill. One man from San Francisco remembers that "as the 80s started...more and more people were getting sick. Fear was gripping the city and the nation. Gay people stopped going out. Nobody knew how it was transmitted and people were afraid."

Because the disease first showed up in LGBTQ+ communities, some people argued that AIDS was a punishment against LGBTQ+ people, proof that their sexual orientation was wrong or immoral. People who developed AIDS were frequently shunned and made to feel ashamed for being sick. As the years passed, however, it became clear that AIDS was a disease that everyone—LGBTQ+ or straight, male or female, old or young—was vulnerable to, and slowly attitudes began to change.

The late Princess Diana of Wales played a big part in changing people's minds about AIDS. During the 1980s and 1990s, she was frequently photographed visiting AIDS patients, hugging children with AIDS, and showing that she wasn't afraid of catching the disease by doing these things. Her support for AIDS charities helped to make people realize that the disease could strike anyone.

After all, the virus that causes AIDS doesn't know or care whether a human body belongs to an LGBTQ+ person or a straight person. Like all microbes, HIV is interested only in reproducing itself.

# DR. BEATRICE HAHN:
# TRACKING THE SOURCE OF AIDS

In 2006, a microbiologist at the University of Alabama named Dr. Beatrice Hahn discovered a virus that infects wild apes in Africa. She named it simian immunodeficiency virus (SIV), because it causes a disease like AIDS in infected chimps. HIV and SIV are so similar, Beatrice was sure that HIV developed from the chimp virus.

For years, Beatrice had been studying captive chimpanzees in labs. She had already found the HIV-like virus in the lab chimps, but to get the scientific community to believe her theory, she needed to prove that the virus existed in the wild. But how?

Turns out the answer was lying on the jungle floor: chimp droppings.

Beatrice scoured the jungles of Cameroon and Tanzania and sure enough, she found SIV in the fresh chimpanzee poop.

So how did SIV turn into HIV? Beatrice thinks she knows: she calls it the "cut hunter theory." Long ago, ahunter killed a chimp. As he was butchering the animal for cooking, he cut himself. Blood from the meat he was handling got into the cut. And along with the blood came SIV, traveling from the infected chimp to the hunter. Once inside its new host, the virus mutated, becoming HIV.

The hunter probably lived in a small, isolated village, so at first the virus didn't spread far. But Beatrice and her team think that eventually someone infected with HIV got on boat heading south down the Congo River to a city. Then the virus was able to spread rapidly.

"The virus ended up in a major metropolitan area, which would either be Kinshasa or Brazzaville," Beatrice told journalists from *National Geographic* magazine in 2007, naming two cities in the Democratic Republic of the Congo. "That's where we believe the AIDS pandemic really started."

AIDS researchers now think that SIV was passed to humans in the 1930s. In 2007 scientists tested a frozen blood sample taken from a man in Kinshasa in 1959. It contained HIV—the earliest example of HIV infection found so far. HIV probably reached North America in 1977, but it wasn't recognized until the early 1980s.

# CHAPTER 8

# A WAKEUP CALL TO THE WORLD

## COVID-19 PANDEMIC, 2020–21

### 7:30 A.M., DECEMBER 30, 2019

The sun was barely up and Dr. Li Wenliang was already on his way to work in Wuhan, China. Patches of fog clung to the wide brown expanse of the Yangtze River, and he could just see the tips of the skyscrapers above the gray mist. In the parks along the river, people were gathering for their morning tai chi exercises. Dr. Li took deep breaths of the cold air as he strode by. Walking to his job at Wuhan Central Hospital helped him focus for the busy day ahead, and these riverside pathways were his favorite route—in the early mornings they were a rare oasis of calm in this city of 11 million people. Wuhan is an important manufacturing center and transportation hub, so its streets were always crowded with cars, trucks, buses, and people.

Just 33 years old, Li Wenliang was already one of the hospital's top ophthalmologists (pronounced off-thuh-mall-uh-justs), or eye doctors. Dr. Li took his work treating diseases of the eyes very seriously, and he often came in early to spend time catching up with the latest medical research before seeing his first patient of the day.

When Li found an interesting new study or report, he'd take a few minutes to share it with his friends from medical school. Even though they were now working at hospitals all across China, the group of more than 150 young doctors kept in touch almost daily over WeChat, the popular Chinese-language social media network. Li enjoyed joining in the lively debates about new treatments and puzzling cases.

As Li approached the hospital's parking lot, he saw it was already jammed with cars and ambulances. Inside, the emergency depart-ment's waiting room was overflowing and the hallways were thronged with patients and white-coated hospital workers. As he threaded his way through the crowds to get to the elevators, Li watched the activity around him.

For several days he'd noticed that the hospital, always humming with energy and crowded with patients, had seemed even busier than usual. At the end of each shift, the doctors and nurses working in the emergency room staggered out, pale with exhaustion. And to Dr. Li, trained to look closely and pay attention to what he saw, they didn't just seem tired—they looked worried.

A few floors up, on the ophthalmology ward where Li worked, things were quieter. He stepped into his office to review the chart for his first patient of the day, but before he could sit down, his phone buzzed in his pocket—a new email. It was a message from the chief of the emergency room, Dr. Ai Fen. She had sent the email to several doctors throughout the hospital, and she had marked it "urgent."

The email described a patient she had treated a few days earlier. He had come to the emergency room complaining of a fever and trouble breathing. An X-ray showed that he had inflammation in his lungs, and she had diagnosed the man with pneumonia. But something didn't sit right with Dr. Ai. She hadn't yet been able to determine what was causing the man's pneumonia, and the pattern of symptoms reminded her of the patients she'd treated in 2003 who had a disease called severe acute respiratory syndrome, or SARS. What had her really worried, though, was what had been happening over the last three days. Since diagnosing that first patient, six more people had turned up in the hospital's emergency room with the same unusual symptoms, and in each case the cause of the pneumonia was unknown. Whatever was causing the first patient's pneumonia, Dr. Ai suspected it was spreading.

Li Wenliang's first patient of the day arrived. The doctor slipped his phone back into his pocket and started to work, but he couldn't stop thinking about what he had just read. He had learned about SARS in medical school, how a respiratory illness caused by a never-before-seen virus had turned into a pandemic. It had started in China, after a virus usually found only in small mammals mutated and began to infect humans. The disease spread quickly to cities across the globe, infecting more than 8,000 people and killing hundreds, all in the space of less than six months. Then, as quickly as it had emerged, SARS had disappeared again. Could the disease have come back?

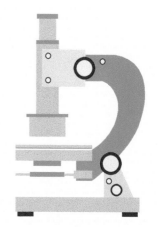

All day long, Li Wenliang asked himself

how he could help fight the danger that had emerged in the emergency room just a few floors below. Was there anything he could do to prevent another epidemic from starting? As a doctor, he had a responsibility to do everything he could to protect people's health against disease.

## 5:30 P.M., DECEMBER 30, 2019

As Li Wenliang said goodbye to his last patient, his mind was made up. He would warn others about what he had learned so that they could protect themselves and their families, and spread the word. He opened WeChat and started typing a message to his group of medical school friends.

"Seven cases of SARS confirmed," Li told the group, and he attached Ai Fen's report on the patient she had examined. He warned his friends that the cases seemed to be connected: according to Ai Fen's email, all the patients either worked at the local Huanan Seafood Market or had shopped there recently. He advised them to take precautions in case another SARS epidemic was beginning, and to tell their families and friends so that they could protect themselves. He pressed Send. For the first time, information about the strange cases of pneumonia in the Wuhan emergency room traveled beyond the hospital's walls.

Li headed for home, eager to see his wife and baby and his parents. And he needed to think about what else he could do to protect others from the risk that a new epidemic might have started in his hospital.

## DECEMBER 31, 2019

Public health scientists in Wuhan sent a report about the cluster of unusual pneumonia cases to China's National Health Commission in Beijing. But with no good information yet on the source of the pneumonia, officials in Wuhan decided it was too soon to say anything to the public about the mysterious cases.

## JANUARY 1, 2020

The Wuhan city government sent police officers to close down the Huanan Seafood Market, the only connection discovered so far between the strange cases of pneumonia turning up in hospital emergency rooms around town. The police ordered all the vendors home, locked the doors, and put up fencing around the outside of the market. They posted guards to make sure shoppers stayed away. Inside, workers in masks and protective gear began scrubbing the building from top to bottom. If something in the market was causing the infection, they hoped that by closing it to the public, the cases of mysterious pneumonia would stop.

## JANUARY 2, 2020

Health officials in Wuhan published information online about the pneumonia cases appearing in the city's hospitals. So far, they said, there was no evidence that whatever was causing the pneumonia outbreak could be spread from person to person, but even so, people should take precautions, like avoiding crowds.

## 1:30 A.M., JANUARY 3, 2020

"Dr. Li! Dr. Li, please answer the door!"

The shouts and knocking at his front door woke Li Wenliang out of a sound sleep. Stumbling out of bed, he forgot to put on his glasses, and when he opened the door, the faces of the police officers were only a hazy blur. But he could tell from their stern tones that there was an urgent reason for this late-night visit. He was in trouble—but for what?

"Are you Dr. Li, the ophthalmologist from the Wuhan Central Hospital?"

"Yes. What do you want at this time of night?"

"You'll need to come with us to the police station. We have some questions to ask you about the rumors that you have been spreading on the internet."

Someone from Li's private WeChat group had shared his post on a public website, and Li's message to his fellow physicians had worried a lot of people. Already there were whispers that a new SARS outbreak was beginning in the city. Before sounding the alarm and making an official announcement, the city government wanted to have more information. Were the pneumonia cases caused by SARS—or by something else? Was the disease contagious, or had the patients all become infected by something at the market? They needed time, and to get that time they needed Li Wenliang to cooperate.

That's why the police arrived at his door. They were there to send him a message: stop talking about the hospital's pneumonia cases.

"You're an eye specialist, right?" The officer in charge shook his head. "What do you know about pneumonia anyway?"

"I can read a medical case report!" Li responded angrily. "And so can the other doctors I sent the report to. They're worried, that's why they've shared my warning online."

"Dr. Li, you need to agree not to publish anything more about these cases. Let the experts study the evidence. If it's SARS, they'll take the proper steps to protect Wuhan."

In the end, Li signed a statement agreeing that he had been wrong to tell others about the pneumonia cases at his hospital. He went back to work and tried to focus on treating his patients. But he was so angry about being told not to talk about the cases in the emergency room that a few days later he posted the statement he'd been forced to sign on Weibo, a Chinese social media site.

Around the city and across the country, concerns grew about the disease outbreak in Wuhan. In the city's laboratories, scientists scrambled to find the cause of the mysterious infection. Meanwhile, doctors cared for the pneumonia patients struggling to breathe, and kept a watchful eye out for signs that the disease was spreading to others.

## JANUARY 3, 2020

Chinese public health officials sent a report to the World Health Organization about the Wuhan pneumonia cases. Already, 44 people in Wuhan had come down with pneumonia symptoms, and doctors hadn't yet been able to identify the cause.

The World Health Organization, or WHO, is an international organization formed by the United Nations that tracks evolving infectious diseases around the world, ready to sound the alarm to protect us all from emerging epidemics. The next day, the WHO tweeted about the cases: "#China has reported to WHO a cluster of #pneumonia cases—with no deaths—in Wuhan, Hubei Province. Investigations are underway to identify the cause of this illness." They told countries around the world to start taking extra precautions against respiratory diseases, and a team of WHO investigators headed to Wuhan to help solve the mystery.

## 11:20 A.M., JANUARY 8, 2020

Li Wenliang bent in close to examine his patient's eye. As he did, she started coughing.

"Oh, excuse me, Doctor. I'm afraid I have a cold. I would have stayed in bed today, but I didn't want to miss my appointment with you," the patient apologized, in between coughs.

"No problem. Now, can you read the letters on the chart against the wall for me?"

Dr. Li continued the examination.

## JANUARY 9, 2020

Doctors in Wuhan fought for the life of a 61-year-old man infected with the mysterious pneumonia. But the infection-fighting medicines, ventilators, and other supports couldn't save him. He died that day, the first victim of the new disease. He had been a regular shopper at the Huanan Seafood Market.

## FINDING THE PANDEMIC'S SOURCE

It didn't take long for doctors to realize that the Huanan Seafood Market was coming up over and over again in their interviews. All of the very first patients either were workers at the market or had shopped there recently. Something at the market was causing the disease—but what?

The Huanan Seafood Market was a large building filled with stalls run by different vendors selling fresh fruit, vegetables, meat, and seafood. Some vendors at the Huanan Seafood Market specialized in selling live wild animals, for food or as pets. Wildlife markets are found all around the world, not only in China, and epidemiologists warn that buying and selling wild animals increases the risk that an animal disease will "make the leap" and infect humans. Animals that wouldn't normally encounter each other in the wild are often brought together at these markets. One animal can pass a virus along to others that have no antibodies against it. Now instead of one sick animal, there are many, and the chances increase that the virus will spread to workers or customers.

While no one knows exactly how the novel coronavirus made the leap to humans, some researchers think that bats were the host species and that it passed from bats to another type of animal and then on to humans at the Huanan Seafood Market.

When Li heard the news, he thought about Dr. Ai Fen and his other friends who worked every day in the emergency wards and the danger they faced. Already the medical staff treating the cases of pneumonia at Wuhan Central Hospital were swathed in protective equipment, and the patients were kept carefully isolated from others. Were those protections enough?

Epidemiologists were kept busy day and night tracking down everyone who had been in contact with one of the pneumonia patients: they needed to know if the disease was spreading, and if so, how fast. The citizens of Wuhan were warned to protect themselves by staying home when they could and wearing masks when out in public. Drugstores quickly ran out of face masks and gloves as people rushed to buy up all they could find.

Meanwhile, the scientists searching for the source of the disease looked anxiously at their calendars: the Lunar New Year was approaching. Every year during this major holiday, millions of people would head out across the country to visit their families. Because Wuhan is a transportation hub, many travelers would be boarding planes, trains, or buses in the city. The scientists knew they needed to determine whether the mysterious illness could be transmitted directly from person to person. If it was contagious, they had to get a warning out in time, or the epidemic could become uncontrollable.

## JANUARY 11, 2020

At last, Chinese scientists found the answer to the question that all of Wuhan was asking: What was causing the outbreak? The source of the illness was a virus in the same family as SARS: a coronavirus. Coronaviruses are named for the way they look, as though each tiny, round virus is wearing a crown (*corona* is the Latin word for crown). Coronaviruses are very common, and they cause diseases in both animals and humans. Most of the human diseases from coronaviruses are mild, like the common cold. But what the scientists had found this time was a completely new virus, one that had never been seen before. Already they knew that it could be lethal.

In the report sent to the WHO and other public health agencies around the world, the scientists referred to their discovery as a "novel" (or new) coronavirus. Not only had they succeeded in identifying the virus, the scientists were able to report that they had already sequenced the genome of the virus. This meant that they had gathered specific information about the virus itself and how it was constructed. Knowing the genetic makeup of the virus would help scientists to develop accurate tests for the mysterious disease. This was crucial in the race to understand the novel coronavirus.

But scientists in China and with the WHO knew there was much more they needed to learn about their new enemy. As they continued to study the disease, they began to put together the picture of what happens inside someone infected with the virus.

# SIGNS AND SYMPTOMS

The novel coronavirus attaches itself to cells in the upper respiratory tract—the parts of the body we use to breathe and speak, such as the nose and throat. That sets off alarm bells for the immune system, which starts to attack the virus. Within a few days, or up to two weeks later, an infected person typically begins to have symptoms of COVID-19: a sore throat, runny nose, fever, and a cough.

Sometimes those symptoms are so mild, the infected person barely notices. But even someone who doesn't feel sick can still infect others. That's part of what makes COVID-19 a difficult disease to control. With other coronavirus infections, like SARS, people got sick very quickly, and as soon as they did they could be isolated so they didn't spread the disease to anyone else.

# TOOL OF THE TRADE:
# STAYING AHEAD OF THE CURVE

As COVID-19 spread, public health officials asked people to help "flatten the curve." An epidemic curve is a tool epidemiologists use to monitor the spread of disease, track down the source of the outbreak, and slow or stop its transmission.

Epidemiologists record the date the first victim became sick on a graph. Then they add each new infection along the y-axis and the number of days since the first case on the x-axis. Drawing a line from point to point creates the curve, and its shape gives scientists important clues about the epidemic. There are three main types of curves:

- **Point source outbreak:** A curve that shoots up suddenly and then drops off shows that many people got sick in a short period of time, with fewer cases occurring each day. That tells the epidemiologists to look for a single source for the outbreak, like contaminated food.

- **Continuous common source epidemic:** A curve that rises to a peak, falls, and then rises slightly tells the epidemiologists there is an ongoing source of contamination. This is the curve that John Snow would have seen for the Broad Street cholera epidemic. When people stopped drinking contaminated water, the curve flattened entirely as the epidemic ended.

- **Progressive source epidemic:** When a disease is spreading from person to person, the epidemic curve shows a series of peaks, each one bigger than the last. Each wave of infection involves more people, until either everyone has been infected or a vaccine is introduced.

## WHAT'S IN A NAME?

Swine Flu or H1N1? AIDS or "Gay-Related Immune Deficiency"? COVID-19 or the "Chinese virus"? The names we use for diseases matter—a lot. If the name of a disease seems to blame a certain region or group, it can lead to finger-pointing. People have experienced discrimination, lost their jobs, and even been threatened. None of it helps protect us or prevent disease.

In 2015, the World Health Organization published guidelines for naming new diseases: no references to people, places, animals, or jobs allowed. Now, when scientists name a new disease, they try to use initials or terms that can't be identified with a specific group of people, to avoid causing discrimination.

Most people who get COVID-19 develop only mild symptoms. But sometimes the virus moves on to invade cells in the lungs, clogging them with inflammation. Patients whose lungs are infected have trouble breathing. The air sacs in the lungs fill with fluid, and not enough oxygen is able to get into the bloodstream from the lungs: pneumonia has set in.

A pneumonia symptom that concerned the doctors in Wuhan who treated the first COVID-19 infections is known as "ground glass" patches. In a CT scan, a COVID-19 patient's lungs are likely to show white patches that may extend right to the edges: pockets of fluid. The Wuhan doctors had seen these patches before, in SARS patients. Both SARS and COVID-19 are caused by coronaviruses. The patches can grow and spread quickly, and patients may need to be given extra oxygen or a ventilator to help them breathe. But a ventilator can't cure the virus: it only helps deliver oxygen, buying more time that may allow the body to fight off the infection.

In patients whose immune systems can't fight the virus, the lungs continue to fill with fluid patches, and eventually their hearts begin to fail. As their blood pressure drops, their bodies go into shock and begin to shut down.

## 7:30 AM, JANUARY 12, 2020

Li Wenliang walked through the doors of the hospital to begin another day of work. He felt hot, light-headed, exhausted. It was hard to breathe.

A nurse rushing by stopped when she saw him. "Dr. Li? You look terrible! Come with me, I'll have someone examine you."

Dr. Li was admitted to the hospital with symptoms of pneumonia later that day. He remembered his patient with the cough. He'd been so focused on the woman's vision problems that he'd forgotten to be concerned about the pathogens she might have been spreading in his small office. Had she recovered from her cold, or had she been suffering from the strange pneumonia-like disease?

As he lay in bed, fighting to breathe and watching the nurses and doctors sheathed in protective masks and suits around him, Li wondered whether the warning he had tried to share on social media would have helped prevent the outbreak from spreading. Scientists were still not convinced that the virus could be spread from person to person, but Li couldn't remember the last time he'd been to the Huanan Seafood Market. He was sure that his illness could be traced back to that eye examination with the coughing patient.

## JANUARY 13, 2020

Thailand reported that a traveler from Wuhan had developed the novel coronavirus, the first case outside China. Scientists from the World Health Organization began to study whether the coronavirus can be transmitted between people.

### JANUARY 16, 2020

Japan confirmed its first case. The WHO sent an international alert, telling countries around the world to start screening air travelers and to take precautions to prevent infection.

### JANUARY 19, 2020

The World Health Organization tweeted that there was evidence that the novel coronavirus could be transmitted from person to person.

### JANUARY 20, 2020

Dr. Zhong Nanshan, China's top epidemiologist, was called in to take charge of the situation in Wuhan. He confirmed on Chinese television that a new virus was causing the illness, that it was spreading between people, and that it appeared to be very contagious. There were now almost 300 confirmed cases in the city.

### JANUARY 23, 2020

Dr. Zhong ordered the city of Wuhan into quarantine to try to stop the spread of the virus. At 10:00 that morning, all buses, trains, and flights coming into or leaving the city were canceled. Subway trains stopped running. Barricades went up on the highways around the city. Schools and businesses were shut down, and people stayed in their homes, only going out for groceries. It was just two days before the Lunar New Year holiday. The officials hoped they had acted in time to contain the virus.

In the days that followed, other cities in China restricted travel; ordered schools, restaurants, and stores to close; and told their citizens to stay home. Cases were appearing around the country, and now they were starting to show up in Hong Kong and in neighboring countries. In China and around the world, scientists were watching and waiting to see if the lockdown could contain the disease, or if it would break out somewhere else.

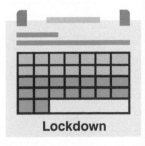

**Lockdown**

# A SCIENCE FAIR PROJECT
# TO CLOSE SCHOOLS

In 2006, Laura Glass was looking for an idea to enter in the annual science fair. With some help from her dad, research scientist Robert Glass, Laura built a computer simulation that showed how people interact during an epidemic. According to Laura's research, kids in school come into contact with more people than any other group: about 140 people every day! That makes closing schools a vital step in controlling epidemics.

Laura's project won third prize at an international science fair—and afterward, the White House called. The U.S. government wanted to hear about the science fair project that showed closing schools could prevent the spread of disease. In 2007, the Centers for Disease Control and Prevention made social distancing and closures of schools and workplaces an official part of the U.S. government's plans for fighting the next pandemic.

## JANUARY 30, 2020

The World Health Organization declared the novel coronavirus a Public Health Emergency of International Concern. That meant they believed the virus presented a serious and sudden health risk, that it might travel across the world, and that international action might be needed to address the threat. Already, 82 cases had been confirmed outside of China. Wuhan's lockdown may have slowed the spread of the epidemic, but it hadn't stopped it.

## FEBRUARY 1, 2020

From his hospital bed, Li started his last post on Weibo: "Today the nucleic acid test result is positive, the dust has settled, and the diagnosis has finally been confirmed." He knew at last what was making him so sick: the new virus that had already killed many others in his city, the virus he had tried to warn others about more than a month ago. He took a selfie and posted it: a pale, exhausted man, his eyes wide and frightened above the respirator covering his face.

There were now more than 10,000 confirmed cases of infections with the novel coronavirus in China.

## FEBRUARY 6, 2020

Wuhan Central Hospital announced that Dr. Li had died. Across China and around the globe, people posted messages on WeChat and Weibo honoring the doctor who had been the first to try to warn the world about the coming epidemic. Many used the hashtag #IWantFreedomofSpeech, calling on their government to stop monitoring and censoring its citizens on social media.

## FEBRUARY 11, 2020.

The World Health Organization declared that the disease caused by the novel coronavirus would be called COVID-19, for "COronaVIrus Disease of 2019."

The Chinese government launched an investigation into why the Wuhan police had told Dr. Li not to share his concerns about the virus. The investigation found that the police should not have told Dr. Li to stay silent. Silence, they agreed, was more dangerous to public health than even the most alarming true information. In an interview on national TV, Dr. Zhong praised Li Wenliang for speaking out. "He's the hero of China," said Zhong, choking back tears. "I'm so proud of him, he told the truth, back in December . . . Honesty is what matters. The public needs to know the truth; concealing what happens may lead to a panic rather than to social stability."

# STOPPING THE INFO-DEMIC

- Eating sea lettuce can prevent you from getting COVID-19. FALSE!

- Mosquitoes spread the coronavirus. FALSE!

- Drinking hot water will wash the virus out of your system. FALSE!

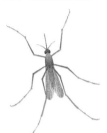

- An easy way to find out if you have COVID-19 is to see if you can hold your breath for more than 10 seconds. FALSE!

- The President of Russia set lions loose in Moscow to convince people to stay inside during the COVID-19 pandemic. FALSE!

During a pandemic, we all want information that will help to keep us safe. Unfortunately, rumors and myths about COVID-19 spread just as fast as the disease itself. Epidemiologists at the World Health Organization soon realized that they had two epidemics to manage: the disease itself and an info-demic that was spreading out of control.

One problem caused by a flood of false information is that people who believe it are less likely to follow the advice of health professionals—and they may do things that put their own lives at risk. Health organizations like the Centers for Disease Control and Prevention and the World Health Organization are fighting back against the fake news info-demic by sharing good information on social media. And everyone has a role to play in slowing down the spread of misinformation, by thinking before sharing a post, and looking for signs that it could be false information.

# THE WHO MISSION

In early February, an international delegation of epidemiologists, led by Dr. Bruce Aylward, traveled to China to study the emergence of COVID-19. They arrived in Wuhan to find a ghost city. The airport and train station were silent and deserted. They drove through empty streets, past shuttered businesses. There were no dog-walkers or joggers on the sidewalks or in the parks. The playgrounds stood empty and still. As the scientists made their way to their hotel, Bruce could sense the tension of 11 million people, waiting inside their homes. Waiting until it was safe to come out.

For 10 days, the scientists traveled to affected cities and towns across China, interviewing hundreds of patients, doctors, nurses, and family members. Their goal was to gather as much information as possible about the virus and how it was transmitted, and to review the measures that were being put in place to prevent the spread of the disease.

At the end of the mission, Bruce congratulated the Chinese government on their efforts to contain the disease with low-cost, low-tech measures like handwashing, mask-wearing, social-distancing, suspending travel, and stay-at-home advisories. He said, "They took this old approach and then turbo-charged it with modern science and modern technology in a way that was unimaginable even a few years ago." The turbo-charging included setting up temperature monitoring stations in public places to quickly scan for people who might have early symptoms of COVID-19, CT scans and testing, contact tracing to identify everyone an infected person might have been in contact with, and quarantine hospitals with special wards to keep patients isolated and medical staff as safe as possible. The WHO delegation estimated that the strategies in Wuhan and other cities across the country had prevented hundreds of thousands of people from becoming infected with COVID-19.

The strategy had worked: they had slowed down the spread of the virus in China. But the infection was already spreading around the world, and countries everywhere were scrambling to keep people safe. Cities went quiet as people stayed inside, waiting for the danger to pass.

Meanwhile, journalists and scientists began to ask questions about exactly how and when the virus emerged. It may be years before scientists put together the full story of where the novel coronavirus came from, when it passed into humans, and how it became such a threat. But the heroes of the story are the brave doctors and scientists working to save lives.

## DON'T PANIC, IT'S A PANDEMIC

When government officials plan for disasters, they wonder: "How will we deal with the public panic?" But in a disaster, many people are more likely to be caring and helpful, even to strangers, than to act selfishly or to panic. The COVID-19 pandemic is no exception.

In Britain, the National Health Service put out a call for volunteers to support elderly people who were isolated because of the pandemic, hoping to get 250,000 volunteers. More than three times that many people responded.

In the province of British Columbia, in Canada, Provincial Health Officer Dr. Bonnie Henry ended her daily pandemic press conferences with the reminder "Be calm, be kind, be safe." By helping people to understand that we must rely on each other, Dr. Henry inspired people in B.C. to act responsibly.

So far, scientists have found a few ways that the virus spreads. When an infected person coughs, sneezes, shouts, or talks without a mask, they release a cloud of droplets that quickly fall to the ground. If someone nearby inhales the droplets, they can be infected. The smallest of the droplets, called aerosols, stay in the air longer, and there is also a risk that people can get infected by breathing them.

# CHOOSE YOUR BATTLE

With a new and dangerous virus infecting more people each day, governments around the world had to act fast to keep people safe.

In Taiwan and South Korea, the governments ordered all businesses to close, except for services that people need to survive. They told everyone to stay home as much as possible. And they introduced high-tech monitoring systems to track those who had come into contact with infected people so they could isolate themselves and prevent further infections. It worked. Infection rates went down. But when businesses re-opened, the number of cases went back up. People began to realize that they would have to take precautions against the virus for a very long time—possibly years.

On the other hand, Swedish public health officials recommended that people avoid large gatherings, keep apart when they could, and wash their hands frequently. But they didn't close businesses or schools, and they didn't require wearing masks. As a result, they had more cases than other countries in Europe during the spring of 2020. But some people think that means that the outbreak in Sweden will end earlier than elsewhere.

We don't know yet which approach will save the most lives. The world is engaged in the biggest science experiment of all time: *Homo sapiens* vs. coronavirus.

Or the droplet lands on a surface, and when someone touches the surface and then brings their hand to their eyes, nose, or mouth, the virus moves in. In most cases, people with COVID-19 only spread the disease to one or two others, if anyone. But in some cases, someone with the disease may infect many others, through what are called "superspreading events." In a superspreading event, lots of people in an enclosed space together are exposed to an infected person at once. Bars, restaurants, prisons, factories, churches, parties—they've all been locations for superspreading.

You might think that superspreading is the coronavirus's superpower. But it's also its weak point. Scientists know that if we can avoid superspreading events, we can lower the transmission rate and stop the epidemic.

As COVID-19 spread around the world in February and March 2020, some people blamed China, saying that the government had been too slow in warning the world and the people of Wuhan. They argued that if people like Dr. Li Wenliang had been allowed to keep posting on social media, the disease might have gotten more attention and people would have known sooner that they needed to protect themselves from catching COVID-19.

We'll never know what difference Dr Li's warning might have made if it had reached more people, or whether earlier information would have prevented some of the infections in Wuhan. But what is certain is that COVID-19, like all human diseases, doesn't stop at borders or recognize the lines we draw on maps to separate one country from another. COVID-19 is an international disease, and it will take an international effort to control its spread. That means working together, sharing what we know so that scientists and doctors have access to the best and most up-to-date information to keep us all safe and healthy.

# FINDING SOMEONE TO BLAME

Early in the pandemic, Dr. Tedros Adhanom Ghebreyesus, the head of the World Health Organization, made a speech calling on the people of the world to work together to fight the disease, instead of blaming one another:

> *The greatest enemy we face is not the virus itself;*
> *it's the stigma that turns us against each other.*
> *We must stop stigma and hate!*
> *We have a choice. Can we come together to face a common*
> *and dangerous enemy? Or will we allow fear, suspicion, and*
> *irrationality to distract and divide us?*
> *This is a time for facts, not fear.*
> *This is a time for rationality, not rumors.*
> *This is a time for solidarity, not stigma.*

Pointing fingers at others and blaming them for spreading infection has a long, sad history. During the Black Plague, Jewish communities were sometimes suspected of starting outbreaks. Because Jewish people were already discriminated against in Europe during the Middle Ages, they were often forced to live together in isolated communities, which weren't hit as hard as the cities were when plague arrived. That led to accusations that Jewish people were responsible for the disease. Jewish people were killed and their communities destroyed because of these rumors.

When people began dying of AIDS in the United States during the 1980s, some feared that people from the island of Haiti were carriers of the disease. Parents refused to let their children go to school if Haitian children were allowed to attend. Haitians were attacked, lost their jobs, and were kicked out of their homes.

# INDIGENOUS STRENGTH
# IN A TIME OF PANDEMIC

Indigenous Peoples in many parts of the world experience racism and oppression that affect their living conditions. They may have trouble accessing medical care, nutritious food, or clean water. Because of discrimination, they might live in crowded conditions or have uncertain sources of income.

For all these reasons, Indigenous people are at a higher risk of suffering from COVID-19. For example, in May 2020, the United Nations reported that people in the Navajo Nation in Arizona were getting sick with COVID-19 at a rate 10 times faster than other people in the state.

Elders and leaders of Indigenous communities are taking action to protect their people, by drawing on their traditional knowledge and healing practices.

In Thailand, the Karen people have revived their ancient ritual of *Kroh Yee* (village closure) to fight the spread of COVID-19. In Morocco, the Amazigh people are using traditional disinfection and purification plants to help prevent the spread of the virus. In Paraguay, elders from the Mbya-Guarani people are sharing their traditional knowledge to make natural disinfectants from local plants.

"The pandemic is a warning," says Lee Maracle, a writer and member of the Sto:lo Nation in Canada. "We need to look at ourselves and our way of life. We have to care for the earth, to preserve what we need to live sustainably."

# CONCLUSION

# PANDEMICS AND THE FUTURE OF DISEASE DETECTION

Way back in 1967, the top doctor in the United States famously declared, "We can now close the book on infectious disease." He believed that the story of epidemics and outbreaks was over, and it had ended with everyone living happily ever after in a disease-free world. When we look back at those words, they seem incredibly optimistic. It is hard to imagine a scientist making that claim today—they'd be more likely to say that we haven't yet finished reading the first chapter on infectious disease.

To be fair, at the time it really did look as if science was winning the war against disease. Vaccination campaigns were wiping out smallpox and polio, diseases that had killed millions in the past. There were good treatments for other feared killer diseases, like tuberculosis. DDT and other pesticides were keeping mosquitoes at bay, so diseases like yellow fever and malaria were no longer such a danger.

More than 50 years later, those diseases that were thought to be gone forever have surged back, resisting the drugs that we once thought had defeated them. Mosquitoes now transmit newly emerged diseases to humans, adding West Nile, Zika, and chikungunya to the list of mosquito-borne viruses that infect humans, along with yellow fever and dengue fever. And now, of course, there is COVID-19, the latest virus to make the leap from animals to humans.

The reasons behind the return of old diseases and the emergence of new diseases are complex. In some cases, we depended too much on the miracle cures of drugs, and forgot simple things, like how washing our hands with soap can take care of many viruses. We pushed back the wilderness at an unprecedented rate, logging forests, building towns and farms, and generally disrupting ecosystems where animals and their microbes had been living together for thousands of years, leaving us largely alone. We looked for others to blame when outbreaks happened, instead of accepting that we are all connected, and that we each have a role and a responsibility in maintaining our collective health and the health of our planet.

At the end of an epidemic or pandemic, after we have been staying home and maintaining social distance, doing our best not to spread a disease that is already endangering our communities, it's natural to wonder: Is it safe to go out again? Is it okay to see friends? Will everything that was closed reopen? Will there be another wave of infections?

Most of all, what we really want to know is: When will everything go back to normal? The short answer is: "When the rate of new infections slows down, flattening the epidemic curve." The clearest way to reach that goal is to vaccinate as many people as possible.

The tough answer is that maybe life will never go back to "normal"—and maybe it shouldn't. COVID-19 started with a virus that lived in an animal, that jumped to a human, that in a matter of weeks spread all around the globe. That should be a wakeup call to the world about how closely we are all linked—viruses, animals, and people. For us to continue to survive, we need to find a way to live in balance with our ecosystem neighbors. The health of human beings is connected to the health of wildlife, and the microbes that they support; when we invade their territory, clearing bush and felling trees to make more room for ourselves, our actions have consequences for our own well-being.

After the last great pandemic, the Spanish flu of 1918, people tried to forget and move on, looking ahead to a new century of progress in which they hoped to defeat disease. Every epidemic and pandemic presents an opportunity to do things a little differently: to remember and to learn from the past.

As you get ready to close this book on infectious diseases, don't imagine that you've heard the last of our friends the microbes. For good and for bad, they're a part of our world, and our future probably holds more new diseases, more epidemics, and even pandemics. And we will continue to depend on disease detectives—both human and wildlife epidemiologists—to help keep us safe.

# GLOSSARY

**ANESTHESIA:** any drug given to patients to take away pain during surgery

**ANTIBODIES:** substances produced by the immune system to defend the body against viruses or bacteria

**ARBOVIRUS:** An acronym for "arthropod-borne virus" to refer to any of a group of viruses that are transmitted by arthropods (animals with exoskeletons, including mosquitoes and ticks). Arboviruses cause diseases in humans such as yellow fever, malaria, and West Nile fever.

**BACTERIA (OR BACTERIUM):** single-celled microscopic organism (plural: bacteria)

**BUBONIC PLAGUE:** most common form of plague, a severe and sometimes fatal bacterial infection caused by flea bites, with symptoms including swollen lymph nodes (called buboes) and fever

**CARRIER:** a person infected with a disease who does not have symptoms but can transmit the disease to others

**CESSPOOL:** underground chamber built to hold sewage, usually from a house

**CONTACT TRACING:** identifying and monitoring people who have been exposed to a disease, to stop the spread of infection

**CORONAVIRUS:** One of a family of viruses that cause illnesses ranging from the common cold to severe acute respiratory syndrome (SARS) and COVID-19. A new strain of coronavirus that has not been seen before in humans is called a "novel coronavirus."

**CYANOSIS:** reaction of the skin to lack of oxygen, causing it to turn blue

**ENDEMIC DISEASE:** a disease regularly found in a certain area or population (e.g., chicken pox and mumps are endemic diseases in North America)

**EPIDEMIC:** a sharp increase in the number of cases of a disease among a large number of people over a wide area

**EPIDEMIOLOGY:** the study of diseases, how they spread, and how they can be controlled

**FECES:** solid bodily waste

**FILOVIRUS:** one of a family of viruses that cause hemorrhagic fevers in humans, including Ebola

**HEMORRHAGIC FEVER:** disease caused by a virus that results in fever and bleeding

**HERD IMMUNITY:** Resistance to the spread of a disease that happens when a large percentage of the population has been either infected or vaccinated. Also called indirect protection.

**IMMUNOLOGY:** the science and study of the immune system, the body's defense against disease

**LAUDANUM:** drug derived from opium, formerly used to treat sickness and sedate patients

**LGBTQ+:** short form for lesbian, gay, bisexual, transgender, and queer

**MIASMA:** vapors formerly thought to contain disease-causing contagion

**MICROBE:** microscopic organism, such as a bacteria or virus, responsible for causing disease

**MORTALITY RATE:** number of deaths in a certain period of time, from a particular cause, in a population (e.g., the mortality rate from car accidents in the U.S. from 1999 to 2005 was 15.4 deaths per 100,000)

**MUTATE:** to change

**OUTBREAK:** a sudden increase in the number of cases of a disease, usually in a small area or among a small group

**PANDEMIC:** global epidemic or series of epidemics of a single disease affecting a large portion of the world at the same time

**PATHOGEN:** an organism that causes disease, such as a virus, bacteria, fungus, or parasite

**PNEUMONIC PLAGUE:** form of plague caused by inhaling infected droplets from another patient, affecting lungs; often fatal

**QUALITATIVE RESEARCH:** the study of behavior through methods such as observation, interviews, and surveys

**QUANTITATIVE RESEARCH:** the study of phenomena using statistical techniques and numerical data

**QUARANTINE:** to keep someone or something apart from others in order to stop the spread of disease; also, the place where people are held while under quarantine

**REHYDRATE:** to restore lost water to the body, such as by drinking water or rehydration fluid

**RESERVOIR SPECIES:** Organisms that host (or harbor) the microbes that cause a particular disease. Usually, the disease does not cause symptoms, or causes only mild symptoms, in the reservoir species (examples are ducks and geese, the reservoir species for avian influenza).

**SANITATION:** keeping living conditions clean in order to maintain health

**SEPTICEMIC PLAGUE:** form of plague in which bacteria invade the bloodstream, causing death

**VACCINE:** medicine that prevents disease by training the body's immune system to fight a disease it has not yet come into contact with

**VIRUS:** Simplest form of germ, visible only under an electron microscope. Viruses cause diseases ranging from influenza and the common cold to yellow fever and AIDS.

**WORKHOUSE:** 19th-century institution for housing the poor

**ZOONOSIS:** a disease that can be transmitted from animals to humans, or from humans to other animals

# WANT TO LEARN MORE?

There are lots of great resources in your local library and online about the history of the diseases described in this book. Check out these suggestions as a starting point for your explorations into the fascinating world of epidemiology:

### EPIDEMIOLOGY

*Epidemiologists: Disease Detectives*. PSB Learning Resources. Go to: https://www.pbslearningmedia.org/resource/envh10.health.lp912/epidemiologists-disease-detectives/.

### PLAGUE

*The Great Plague and Fire of London* by Charles J. Shields. Philadelphia, PA: Chelsea House, 2002.

*The Plague* by Holly Cefrey. New York, NY: Rosen, 2001.

### CHOLERA

*The Blue Death: The True Story of a Terrifying Epidemic* by Judy Allen. London, U.K.: Hodder, 2001.

*Cholera: Curse of the Nineteenth Century* by Stephanie True Peters. New York, NY: Marshall Cavendish, 2005.

### YELLOW FEVER

*The Secret of the Yellow Death: A True Story of Medical Sleuthing* by Suzanne Jurmain. Boston, MA: Houghton Mifflin, 2009.

### TYPHOID

"The Most Dangerous Woman in America." An episode of the *NOVA* TV series, PBS, 2004. Go to: https://www.imdb.com/title/tt0662644/.

*You Wouldn't Want to Meet Typhoid Mary!: A Deadly Cook You'd Rather Not Know* by Jacqueline Morley. New York, NY: Franklin Watts/Scholastic Inc., 2013.

### SPANISH INFLUENZA

*The 1918 Influenza Pandemic* by Stephanie True Peters. New York, NY: Marshall Cavendish, 2005.

"Influenza 1918." An episode of the *American Experience* TV series, PBS, 1998. Go to: https://www.pbs.org/video/american-experience-influenza-1918.

## EBOLA

*Ebola* by Aubrey Stimola. New York, NY: Rosen, 2011.

"Ebola—The Plague Fighters." An episode of the *NOVA* TV series, PBS, 1996. Go to: https://www.pbs.org/wgbh/nova/teachers/programs/2304_ebola.html.

*World's Worst Germs: Micro-organisms and Disease* by Anna Claybourne. Chicago, IL: Raintree, 2006.

## AIDS

*AIDS and HIV: The Facts for Kids* by Rae Simons. Vestal, NY: Alphahouse, 2009.

*AIDS: In Search of a Killer* by Suzanne LeVert. New York, NY: Julian Messner, 1987.

*Heroes Against AIDS* by Anna Forbes. New York, NY: PowerKids Press, 1996.

## COVID-19

*Coping with COVID-19. A Pandemic through a Girl's Eyes: 16 adolescent Girls from Nine Countries Film Their Lives under Lockdown.* UNICEF, 2020. Go to: https://www.unicef.org/coronavirus/coping -with-covid-19

"Coronavirus disease (COVID-19) advice for the public: Mythbusters." World Health Organization. Go to: https://www.who.int/emergencies /diseases/novel-coronavirus-2019/advice-for-public/myth-busters.

*How Teenagers Can Protect their Mental Health During Coronavirus COVID-19: 6 strategies for Teens Facing a New (Temporary) Normal.* By UNICEF, 2020. Go to: https://www.unicef.org/coronavirus/how -teenagers-can-protect-their-mental-health-during-coronavirus -covid-19

# SOURCES

## GENERAL

Balzer, Deb. "Pandemic vs. Endemic vs. Outbreak: Terms to Know." *Mayo Clinic*, March 20, 2016. https://newsnetwork.mayoclinic.org/discussion/pandemic-versus-endemic-versus-outbreak-terms-to-know/.

Diamond, Jared. *Guns, Germs, and Steel: The Fates of Human Societies*. New York, NY: W.W. Norton, 1997.

Farrell, Jeanette. *Invisible Enemies: Stories of Infectious Disease*. Second Edition, Revised and Updated. New York, NY: Farrar, Straus Giroux, 2005.

Government of Canada. "Field Epidemiologists: Disease Detectives of Public Health." *The Science of Health* (blog), last modified April 20, 2018. https://www.ic.gc.ca/eic/site/063.nsf/eng/97581.html.

Honigsbaum, Mark. *The Pandemic Century: One Hundred Years of Panic, Hysteria, and Hubris*. New York, NY: W.W. Norton, 2019.

Kahn, Laura H. "A 1947 Smallpox Outbreak Was a 'Textbook Example of a Strong, Humane, and Effective Public Health Response'" *Mother Jones*, April 4, 2020. https://www.motherjones.com/politics/2020/04/this-1947-smallpox-outbreak-was-a-textbook-example-of-a-strong-humane-and-effective-public-health-response/.

Microbiology Society. "Viruses." https://microbiologysociety.org/why-microbiology-matters/what-is-microbiology/viruses.html.Shah, Sonia. *Pandemic: Tracking Contagions, from Cholera to Ebola and Beyond*. New York, NY: Farrar, Straus and Giroux, 2016.

Solnit, Rebecca. *A Paradise Built in Hell: The Extraordinary Communities That Arise in Disaster*. New York, NY: Penguin Group, 2009.

Yong, Ed. *I Contain Multitudes: The Microbes Within Us and a Grander View of Life*. New York, NY: HarperCollins, 2016.

## PLAGUE

Boyce, Niall. "Bills of Mortality: tracking Disease in Early Modern London." *The Lancet 395, no. 10231 (April 2020)*: 1186-87. https://doi.org/10.1016/S0140-6736(20)30725-X.

Carmody, John. "John Graunt and the Birth of Medical Statistics." https://doi.org/10.1016/S0140-6736(20)30725-X. *Ockham's Razor* (podcast). Hosted by Robyn Williams, produced by Brigitte Seega. Australian Broadcasting Corporation (ABC) National Radio. Audio, 12:50. https://www.abc.net.au/radionational/programs/ockhamsrazor/john-graunt-and-the-birth-of-medical-statistics/4279242#transcript.

Cunningham, Kevin. *Diseases in History: Plague*. Greensboro, NC: Morgan Reynolds Publishing, 2009.

Graunt, John. *Reflections on the weekly bills of mortality for the cities of London and Westminster, and the places adjacent: but more especially, so far as it relates to the plague, and other most mortal diseases that we English-men are most subject to, and should be most careful against, in this our age*. London: Printed for Samuel Speed, at the Rainbow in Fleet-Street, 1665. Houghton Library, Harvard University, Cambridge, MA. Accessed at: http://nrs.harvard.edu/urn-3:FHCL.HOUGH:1267760.

Greenberg, S. J. "The Dreadful Visitation: Public Health and Public Awareness in Seventeenth-Century London." *Bulletin of the Medical Library Association 85, no. 4 (October 1997)*: 391–401.

Moote, A. Lloyd, and Dorothy C. Moote. *The Great Plague: The Story of London's Most Deadly Year*. Baltimore, MD: John Hopkins University Press, 2004.

Porter, Stephen. *The Great Plague*. Stroud, U.K.: Sutton Publishing, 1999.

Pryor, E. G. "The Great Plague of Hong Kong." *Journal of the Hong Kong Branch of the Royal Asiatic Society 15 (1975)*: 61–70.

Rothman, Kenneth J. "Lessons from John Graunt." *The Lancet 347 (January 1996)*: 37–39. Accessed at: https://www.sjsu.edu/faculty/gerstman/eks/RothmanArticleOnGraunt1996.pdf.

Stephan, Ed. "John Graunt (1620–1674)." Web database on Graunt's work, https://www.edstephan.org/Graunt/graunt.html.

## CHOLERA

Allen, Judy. *The Blue Death: The True Story of a Terrifying Epidemic*. London: Hodder, 2001.

Badger, Emily. "We've Been Looking at the Spread of Global Pandemics All Wrong." *Bloomberg CityLab.*, February 25, 2013. https://www.bloomberg.com/news/articles/2013-02-25/we-ve-been-looking-at-the-spread-of-global-pandemics-all-wrong.

Hempel, Sandra. *The Strange Case of the Broad Street Pump: John Snow and the Mystery of Cholera.* Berkeley, CA: University of California Press, 2007.

Johnson, Steven. *The Ghost Map: The Story of London's Most Terrifying Epidemic—and How It Changed Science, Cities, and the Modern World.* New York, NY: Riverhead Books, 2006.

Muench, Susan Bandoni. The Mystery of the Blue Death: A Case Study in Epidemiology and the History of Science. *Journal of College Science Teaching* 39, no. 1 (September 2009): 60–66.

Peters, Stephanie True. *Cholera: Curse of the Nineteenth Century.* New York, NY: Marshall Cavendish, 2005.

Sample, Ian. "ClickClinica: the App That Maps Disease Outbreaks." *The Guardian*, November 26, 2012. https://www.guardian.com/science/blog/2012/nov/26/clickclinica-app-map-disease-outbreaks.

UN News. Haiti Cholera Outbreak "Stopped in Its Tracks." January 24, 2020. https://news.un.org/en/story/2020/01/1056021.

## YELLOW FEVER

Agramonte, Aristides. The Inside History of a Great Medical Discovery. *The Scientific Monthly* 1, no. 3 (December 1915): 209–37. Accessed at: https://www.jstor.org/stable/6065.

Altman, Lawrence K. *Who Goes First?: The Story of Self-Experimentation in Medicine.* New York, NY: Random House, 1987.

Dickerson, James L. *Yellow Fever: A Deadly Disease Poised to Kill Again.* Amherst, NY: Prometheus Books, 2006.

Jurmain, Suzanne. *The Secret of the Yellow Death: A True Story of Medical Sleuthing.* Boston, MA: Houghton Mifflin, 2009.

McCullough, David. The Path Between the Seas: The Creation of the Panama Canal, 1870–1914. NY: Simon and Schuster, 1977.

World Health Organization. *A Global Strategy to Eliminate Yellow Fever Epidemics (EYE) 2017–2026.* Geneva, 2018. Accessed at: https://apps.who.int/iris/bitstream/handle/10665/272408/9789241513661-eng.pdf?ua=1.

## TYPHOID

Bourdain, Anthony. *Typhoid Mary: An Urban Historical.* New York, NY: Bloomsbury, 2001.

Leavitt, Judith Walzer. *Typhoid Mary: Captive to the Public's Health.* Boston, MA: Beacon Press, 1996.

Parry, Manon S. "Sara Josephine Baker (1873–1945)." *American Journal of Public Health* 96, no. 4 (April 2006): 620–21.

## SPANISH INFLUENZA

Barry, John M. *The Great Influenza: The Story of the Deadliest Pandemic in History.* NY: Penguin, 2004.

Cohan, George M. "Over There." Audio recordings, performed by Billy Murray, 1917; Nora Bayes, 1917; and Enrico Caruso, 1918. Accessed at: https://www.firstworldwar.com/audio/overthere.htm.

Crosby, Alfred W. *America's Forgotten Pandemic: The Influenza of 1918.* Cambridge, U.K.: Cambridge University Press, 2003.

Daniel, Thomas M. *Wade Hampton Frost, Pioneer Epidemiologist, 1880–1938: Up to the Mountain.* Rochester, NY: University of Rochester Press, 2004.

Duncan, Kirsty. *Hunting the 1918 Flu: One Scientist's Search for a Killer Virus.* Toronto, ON: University of Toronto Press, 2003.

Frost, Wade Hampton. "The Epidemiology of Influenza." *Journal of the American Medical Association* 73 (August 1919): 313–18.

Peters, Stephanie True. *The 1918 Influenza Pandemic.* New York, NY: Marshall Cavendish, 2005.

## EBOLA

Branswell, Helen, 'Against all Odds': The Inside Story of How Scientists across Three Continents Produced an Ebola Vaccine." STAT, January 7, 2020. https://www.statnews.com/2020/01/07/inside-story-scientists-produced-world-first-ebola-vaccine/.

Centers for Disease Control and Prevention. Zombie Preparedness. Accessed at: https://www.cdc.gov/cpr/zombie/index.htm.

Close, William T. *Ebola: Through the Eyes of the People.* Marbleton, WY: Meadowlark Springs Productions, 2002.

Laurie Garrett. *The Coming Plague: Newly Emerging Diseases in a World Out of Balance.* New York, NY: Penguin, 1995.

Piot, Peter, and Michel Sidibé. "A Conversation with Peter Piot." Presided by Laurie Garrett, Council on Foreign Relations. Audio recording, 1:05:00. https://www.cfr.org/event/conversation-peter -piot.

Lovgren, Stefan. "Where Does Ebola Hide Between Epidemics?" *National Geographic News.*

Piot, Peter. *No Time to Lose: A Life in Pursuit of Deadly Viruses.* New York, NY: W.W. Norton & Co., 2012.

Plummer, Francis A., and Steven M. Jones. "The story of Canada's Ebola Vaccine". *CMAJ: Canadian Medical Association Journal* 189, no. 43 (October 2017): E1326–E1327. *https://doi.org/10.1503/cmaj.170704.*

"Robert Koch, 1843–1910." Under "Notable People," *Contagion: Historical Views of Diseases and Epidemics* (exhibit). Harvard Library's Open CollectionsProgram, 2008. Updated in 2020 as part of the CURIOSity Digital Collections. https://curiosity.lib.harvard.edu/ contagion/feature/robert-koch-1843-1910.

Robert Koch Institut. "First Contact: Scientists from the Robert Koch Institute Reconstruct the Origin of the West African Ebola Virus Epidemic." https://www.rki.de/EN/Content/infections /epidemiology/outbreaks/Ebola_virus_disease/Investigative _work/first_contact.html.

Ross, Will. "Ebola crisis: How Nigeria's Dr. Adadevoh Fought the Virus." BBC News, October 20, 2014. https://www.bbc.com/news/world -africa-29696011.

Shah, Sonia, "The Spread of New Diseasesand the Climate Connection," *Yale Environment 360.* October 15, 2009. https://e360.yale.edu /features/the_spread_of_new_diseases_the_climate_connection.

Smith, Tara C. *Ebola: Deadly Diseases and Epidemics* series. Philadelphia, PA: Chelsea House Publishers, 2005.

Stimola, Aubrey. *Ebola.* New York, NY: Rosen Publishing, 2011.

Sureau, P., P. Piot, et al. "Containment and Surveillance of an Epidemic of Ebola Virus Infection in Yambuku Area, Zaire, 1976." In *Proceedings of an International Colloquium on Ebola Virus Disease and Other Haemorrhagic Fevers held in Antwerp, Belgium, 6–8 December, 1977.* Edited by S. R. Pattyn. Amsterdam: Elsevier/North-Holland Biomedical Press, 1978.

## AIDS

Brown, David. "The Emergence of a Deadly Disease." *Washington Post*, June 5, 2001. Accessed at: https://www.washingtonpost.com/wp-dyn/content/article/2006/06/03/AR2006060300452.html.

Epidemic Intelligence Service (EIS) webpages. Centers for Disease Control and Prevention website. www.cdc.gov/EIS/index.html.

Fan, Hung Y., Ross F. Conner, and Luis P. Villarreal. *AIDS: Science and Society*. 7th ed. Burlington, MA: Jones & Bartlett, 2014.

Fee, Elizabeth, and Theodore M. Brown. "Michael S. Gottlieb and the Identification of AIDS." *American Journal of Public Health* 96, no. 6 (June 2006): 982–83. https://doi.org/10.2105/AJPH.2006.088435.

Fisher, Max. "The Story of AIDS in Africa." *The Atlantic*, December 1, 2011. https://www.theatlantic.com/international/archive/2011/12/the-story-of-aids-in-africa/249361/.

Kinsella, James. *Covering the Plague: AIDS and the American Media*. New Brunswick, NJ: Rutgers University Press, 1989.

Knox, Richard. "Epicenter of AIDS Is Found: Africa, 1930." May 25, 2006, in *All Things Considered* (radio program), National Public Radio,. Audio, 4:47. https://www.npr.org/transcripts/5431256.

LeVert, Suzanne. *AIDS: In Search of a Killer*. New York, NY: Julian Messner, 1987.

Owen, James. "AIDS Origin Traced to Chimp Group in Cameroon." National Geographic News, May 25, 2006.

Shilts, Randy. *And the Band Played On: Politics, People, and the AIDS Epidemic*. New York, NY: St. Martin's Press, 1987.

## COVID-19

Fleming, Nic. "Coronavirus Misinformation, and How Scientists Can Help to Fight It." *Nature*. https://www.nature.com/articles/d41586-020-01834-3.

Green, Andrew. "Li Wenliang." *The Lancet* 395, no 10225 (February 29, 2020) https://doi.org/10.1016/S0140-6736(20)30382-2.

Maron, Dina Fine. "'Wet Markets' Likely Launched the Coronavirus. Here's What You Need to Know" *National Geographic*, April 15, 2020. https://www.nationalgeographic.com/animals/2020/04/coronavirus-linked-to-chinese-wet-markets/.

Qiu, Jane. "Chasing Plagues." *Scientific American* 322, no 6, (June 2020) https://doi.org/10.1038/scientificamerican0620-24.

United Nations Department of Economic and Social Affairs. Policy Brief: "The Impact of COVID-19 on Indigenous Peoples." Accessed at: https://www.un.org/development/desa/dpad/wp-content/uploads /sites/45/publication/PB_70.pdf.

United Nations Human Rights, Office of the High Commissioner. "COVID-19 and Indigenous People's Rights: What Is the Impact of COVID-19 on Indigenous Peoples' Rights?" Accessed at: https://www.ohchr.org/Documents/Issues/IPeoples /OHCHRGuidance_COVID19_IndigenouspeoplesRights.pdf.

Waltner-Toews, David. *On Pandemics: Deadly Diseases from Bubonic Plague to Coronavirus.* Vancouver, BC: Greystone Books, 202

# IMAGE CREDITS

Cover illustration (doctor with medical mask): © Lightspring / Shutterstock.com

Cover, 22, 26, 28, 34, 44, 48, 62, 64, 77, 93, 97, 100, 106, 112, 114, 117, 137, 138, 144, 179 BACTERIUMS patterns & illustrations © Nastya Tkachova via CreativeMarket

1, 2, 4, 5, 11, 59, 70, 78, 87, 88, 96, 98, 108, 113, 115, 122, 123, 126, 127, 134, 135, 141, 148, 153, 155, 159, 161, 165, 166, 167, 168, 173, 177, 178 Corona Virus - Flat Vector Icons © Jumbo Icons via CreativeMarket

10, 46, 52, 60, 67 Pest control set with insects © Vector Tradition via CreativeMarket

13, 16, 20 50 Funeral Flat Multicolor Icons © IconBunny via CreativeMarket

14 Guill Feather Pen and Inkwell © TopVectors via CreativeMarket

24, 43, 80 Pharmaceutical apothecary elements set © Shanvood via CreativeMarket

25 Contours and silhouettes Puzzle © LineworkStock via CreativeMarket

29, 169 Disinfection, pest control © Vector Tradition via CreativeMarket

39, 40, 75 Cartoon smoke. Vfx comic bang clouds © Onyx via CreativeMarket

54 Anchor Isolated on White © Shanvood via CreativeMarket

55 Set of military camouflage helmets in khaki camo-colors © Shanvood via CreativeMarket

56 Thermometers. Hospital medical © Onyx via CreativeMarket

67 Butterfly net © studiostoks via CreativeMarket

75 Vector milk bottles © Ruliz via CreativeMarket

84 Icons set, Happy Halloween © studiogstock via CreativeMarket

89 Set of bugles of different colors © Shanvood via CreativeMarket

92 Cereal porridge breakfast Woters via CreativeMarket

110 Chickens flat vector illustration © Yayasya via CreativeMarket

119 Male Soccer Player Kicking Ball © TopVectors via CreativeMarket

125 Monkey icon set, cartoon style © Ylivdesign via CreativeMarket

# INDEX